Politics and Development in Co

Published by one of the world's lea
'Politics and Development in Conte
accessible but in-depth analysis of ke, ~~..~...puia1y issues affecting
countries within the continent. Featuring a wealth of empirical material and case study detail, and focusing on a diverse range of subject
matter – from conflict to gender, development to the environment
– the series is a platform for scholars to present original and often
provocative arguments. Selected titles in the series are published in
association with the International African Institute.

Already published:

Mobility between Africa, Asia and Latin America: Economic Networks and Cultural Interactions, edited by Ute Röschenthaler and Alessandro Jedlowski

Agricultural Development in Rwanda: Authoritarianism, Markets and Spaces of Governance, Chris Huggins

Liberia's Female Veterans: War, Roles and Reintegration, Leena Vastapuu and Emmi Nieminen

Food Aid in Sudan: A History of Power, Politics and Profit, Susanne Jaspars

Kakuma Refugee Camp: Humanitarian Urbanism in Kenya's Accidental City, Bram J. Jansen

Development Planning in South Africa: Provincial Policy and State Power in the Eastern Cape, John Reynolds

Uganda: The Dynamics of Neoliberal Governance, edited by Jörg Wiegratz, Giuliano Martiniello and Elisa Greco

Forthcoming titles:

Negotiating Public Services in the Congo: State, Society and Governance, edited by Kristof Titeca and Tom De Herdt

About the author

Isak Niehaus currently teaches anthropology at Brunel University London. He studied at the universities of Cape Town and the Witwatersrand and has done extensive fieldwork on the topics of witchcraft, sexuality and politics in South African rural areas. Niehaus's previous monographs include *Witchcraft, Power and Politics: exploring the occult in the South African lowveld* (2001) and *Witchcraft and a Life in the New South Africa* (2013).

Published in association with the International African Institute

The principal aim of the International African Institute is to promote scholarly understanding of Africa, notably its changing societies, cultures and languages. Founded in 1926 and based in London, it supports a range of publications including the journal *Africa*. www.internationalafricaninstitute.org

AIDS in the Shadow of Biomedicine

Inside South Africa's Epidemic

Isak Niehaus

ZED

In association with the
International African Institute

AIDS in the Shadow of Biomedicine: Inside South Africa's Epidemic
was first published in 2018 by Zed Books Ltd, The Foundry,
17 Oval Way, London SE11 5RR, UK.

www.zedbooks.net

Typeset in Plantin MT by seagulls.net
Index by Isak Niehaus
Cover design by Keith Dodds
Cover photo © Chris de Bode/Panos

A catalogue record for this book is available from the British Library

ISBN 978-1-78699-473-8 hb
ISBN 978-1-78699-474-5 pb
ISBN 978-1-78699-475-2 pdf
ISBN 978-1-78699-476-9 epub
ISBN 978-1-78699-477-6 mobi

I dedicate this study to the memory of Eliazaar ('Professor') Mohlala, a former primary school teacher and preacher of the Zion Christian Church (ZCC). Eliazaar worked as my assistant for 27 years and played a pivotal role in all phases of research. He died suddenly and unexpectedly, before he could witness the fruits of our joint work in the production of this monograph.

Contents

Map 1. North Eastern South Africa

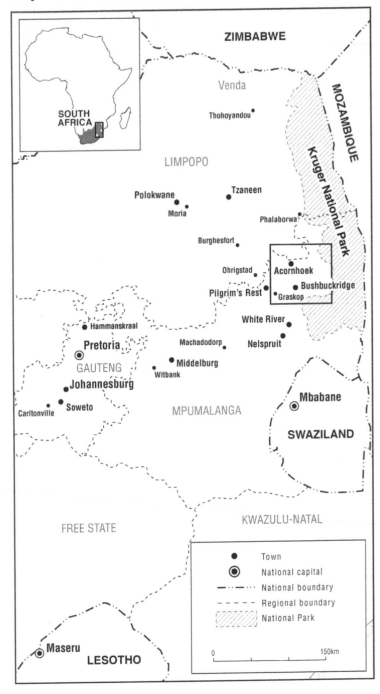

Map 2. The Bushbuckridge Municipality

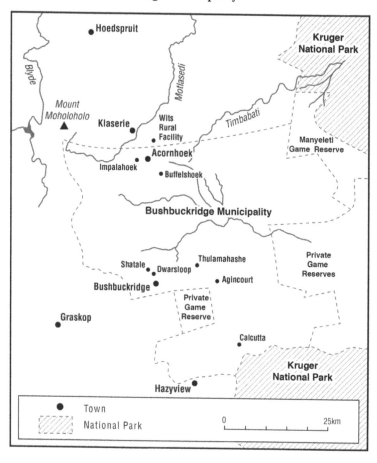

Preface and acknowledgements

At the time of South Africa's first democratic election in 1994, I was in my fourth year of doing fieldwork in Impalahoek,[1] a village populated by nearly 20,000 Northern Sotho and Tsonga[2] speakers, in the country's north-eastern lowveld. Instead of the conventional year in the field, my research was broken up into shorter visits of between one and three months, spread around non-teaching periods at the universities where I worked. Until then, Impalahoek had formed part of Mapulaneng, a region of Lebowa, a relatively impoverished Bantustan. Villagers eagerly anticipated the benefits that a black majority government might bring.

In April 1994, thousands of people flocked to the Thulumahashe stadium, 15 kilometres away, to listen to Nelson Mandela, who led the ANC's (African National Congress's) election campaign. The legendary statesman displayed little euphoria, but in a fatherly manner called upon everyone to play their part in building a new nation. He asked the youth to respect their chiefs, and chiefs to reject tribalism. But his sternest warning was to promiscuous men. There was now a terrible new disease called AIDS, he said, and men who cheated their wives with younger women courted death. Never had any listener heard an elderly man speak so openly about sex in a public forum.

The elections were remarkably calm, and Mandela's party secured a huge majority. Over the next two decades, the ANC-led government sought to ameliorate some of the worst scars of racial oppression. Local government was transferred to the Bushbuckridge municipality and (eventually) also to Mpumalanga Province. During each of my successive visits to the field I saw tangible signs of 'development'. Soon, there was a major shopping centre on the outskirts of the village, and by 1998 the government had issued 1,500 three-roomed houses – with electricity, sanitation and on-site taps – to households earning less than R500 per month. The new municipal and provincial governments provided employment for the poor; issued lucrative service-provision contracts to emerging businesspeople; and oversaw the building of tarred roads and the construction of huge mast lights that formed part of crime prevention operations. South Africa's national government drastically improved social welfare by increasing old age and disability pensions, establishing school feeding schemes, and introducing child maintenance and foster grants.

But democracy also brought new hardships, notably in the form of de-industrialisation and the HIV/AIDS pandemic. Throughout the 1990s, thousands of men, who had previously worked as oscillating migrant labourers in mines and factories on the Witwatersrand, were made redundant.[3] The disease about which Nelson Mandela had warned also arrived. During 1995, Joyce Nkuna, a teacher, showed a pamphlet to her colleagues and to me in the staffroom of the Impalahoek primary school. Its anonymous author(s) claimed that all policemen at the nearest station were HIV-positive and intentionally spread the virus by engaging in unprotected sex with local women. Some teachers doubted whether the allegations were true, and I personally saw them as akin to witchcraft accusations. They articulated well-established tensions between village residents and the police, who had, in earlier years, unscrupulously enforced the repressive laws of the apartheid state. Despite our misgivings, there were soon signs of fatal illness in most residential sections of Impalahoek. Sero-prevalence rates among women receiving ante-natal care at Tintswalo hospital increased from 2 per cent in 1992 to 21 per cent in 2006 and 32 per cent in 2008 (MacPherson et al. 2008: 590).

Only gradually did I begin to learn about the multi-stranded perceptions and experiences of AIDS in the village setting. Since 1990, my research assistants and I had studied witchcraft beliefs and accusations in newly emerging political and economic contexts (Niehaus et al. 2001), the politics of national liberation movements, ethnicity, sexuality and rumours of ritual murder (Niehaus 1993; 2000a; 2000b; 2002a), as well as taboos, concepts of the body, and *muchongolo* dancing (Niehaus 2002b; Niehaus and Stadler 2004). But, while researching other topics, I constantly heard talk of the 'dreaded disease', known through a unique constellation of symptoms: weight loss, diarrhoea, hair loss, coughing, dark sores, discolouration of the mouth, and dementia in the final stages of sickness. Few families were able to escape the debilitating effects of the pandemic. During 2004, the disease intruded into my personal social network, when my research assistant and friend Jimmy Mohale suffered acute attacks of pneumonia. Against the advice of kin and acquaintances, Jimmy refused to test for HIV antibodies,[4] and consulted diviners and Christian healers with the money I had given him in order to seek biomedical treatment. Jimmy died in 2005, convinced that he was a victim of his own father's witchcraft (Niehaus 2013).

Shaken by Jimmy's death, I began to collect information directly about HIV and AIDS in Impalahoek, with the hope that such material might advance scholarly understandings of the pandemic. During my annual visits to Impalahoek during winter vacations, I still conducted participant observation and recorded information about other significant happenings. But I also befriended AIDS activists and home-based carers, attended AIDS awareness workshops, and documented discussions about the reasons for death at the funerals that I attended. With the help of research assistants, I recorded the sexual biographies of 52 men and women, and listened attentively to their personal understandings of HIV and AIDS. Later, as Highly Active Antiretroviral Treatment (HAART) became available, we interviewed persons who had tested positive for HIV antibodies and visited households that fostered AIDS orphans.

During the research process, I began to read and think critically about the dominant theoretical assumptions that guide social scientific literature on the pandemic and found these to diverge starkly from the perspectives of research participants. Appadurai's (1996) analysis of globalisation and Foucault's (1973; 1977), Agamben's (1998; 2005) and Rose's (2001; 2006) works on biopolitics have inspired recent anthropological writings on HIV/AIDS. On the one hand, scholars focus on the transnational flows of pathogens, biomedical concepts and resources deployed to ameliorate the effects of the pandemic. On the other, they make extensive reference to new forms of 'citizenship', in which individuals claim rights to services and support based on their belonging to biomedical categories (Petryna 2002; 2004). Hence, scholars claim, the HIV/AIDS pandemic has given rise to zones of inclusion and exclusion, and to differences between those who live pharmaceutically, and those who do not (Biehl 2006; 2007). In the case of West Africa, Nguyen (2010) shows how people fashion the self through participation in health programmes to gain access to networks of resources and sociality. In a similar vein, social scientists examine how activism by the South African Treatment Action Campaign (TAC) for access to free antiretroviral medication has forged new subjectivities and modes of belonging.

While transnational flows and new forms of 'bio-sociality' might well be crucial, such a focus obscures an understanding of diversities, differences and specificities in the life worlds of people living with AIDS. The diffusion of biomedical understandings of HIV and AIDS seldom possess a linear character. Their flows are more likely to encounter obstacles, and to overlap or intersect with alternative, sometimes competing, perspectives and relationships. This is particularly true of village settings such as Impalahoek, where urban-based activist movements such as TAC have no presence. Here, in a situation marked by critical shortages of clinical resources and by thriving traditions of medical pluralism, the authority of biomedicine is less secure. Prince (2013: 6) observes, in African village settings, that biomedicine 'co-exists with other epistemologies and practices that locate health and therapy in arenas beyond the biological body, outside the clinic and hospital, and among non-biological authorities'.

In this book, I aim to demonstrate the significance of social forms and symbolic meanings that exist in the proverbial 'shadow' of biomedicine for understanding the specificities of people's experiences of HIV/AIDS in Impalahoek. I contend that popular meanings and metaphors of dying and death have contributed to the construction of AIDS as a highly stigmatised condition, that notions of witchcraft have shaped the allocation of blame, and that people's fear of dangerous words and of indiscreet speech have inhibited their inclination to undergo tests for HIV antibodies. I also aim to show how gravely sick people sought to negotiate therapy in contexts of radical health pluralism, confronted diverse aetiologies of disease, and encountered various kinds of healers. Moreover, I suggest that popular understandings of dreams form the backdrop to people's interpretations of the effects of antiretroviral medication, and that vernacular models of kinship, which imply a diffusion of parenthood, have enabled orphans to secure guardianship in the aftermath of AIDS.

This monograph has both scholarly and activist intentions. From an anthropological viewpoint, I reaffirm the contention that global flows have not eradicated pluralism. From a polemical viewpoint, I challenge the adequacy of reductionist, universal notions of sickness that underlie interventions by centrist health bureaucracies in sick people's lives. I suggest that engagement with 'vectors from below' and the empowerment of carers who work directly with the sick in village settings are prerequisites for the more effective provision of more contextually appropriate healthcare.

Historians of anthropology have long exposed the myth of the lone researcher and have shown how the production of anthropological knowledge is essentially a collaborative enterprise (Schumaker 2001; Bank and Bank 2013). My research and writing involved participation in cross-cutting social networks. I could not have completed this work without the help of my research assistants – Eliazaar Mohlala,

Jane Ndlovu and Eric Thobela – and without the involvement of hundreds of research participants who kindly welcomed me into their homes and narrated deeply personal stories to me. Because many of the topics we discussed are of a sensitive nature, I anonymise the identities of all research participants and refer to them only by pseudonyms. This does not diminish my gratitude to them. In the text I have translated their speech from Northern Sotho and Tsonga, and have edited quotations for grammatical inconsistencies when given in English. But I have not sought to censor their voices. In the context of a devastating pandemic, silence might well be a more serious abuse of academic responsibility than the presentation of unpalatable information. Unless specified otherwise, all non-English words in the text are in the Sepulana dialect of Northern Sotho.

I thank Sharon Pollard, Kevin Mitchell and Vusi Dlamini for their hospitality, and the staff of the Wits Rural Facility for providing me with accommodation. My thoughts have been shaped in conversations with Nic Argenti, Liana Chua, Harri Englund, Federica Guglielmo, Elizabeth Hull, Gunvor Jonsson, Stephanie Kitchen, Adam Kuper, Jean La Fontaine, Eva Lukshaite, Brigida Marovelli, James Staples and Giorgia Tresca (in the United Kingdom); Leslie Bank, Mary Crewe, Conny Mathebula, Fraser McNeill, Jimmy Pieterse, John Sharp, Enos Sikhauli, Jonathan Stadler, Robert Thornton, Kees Van der Waal, Rehanna Vally, Charles Van Onselen and Ilana Van Wyk (in South Africa); Erik Bähre (Leiden); Alexander Boscovic (Belgrade); Sylvia de Faveri (Vienna); Fred Golooba-Mutebi (Kampala); Robert Gordon (Vermont); Don Handelman (Jerusalem); Peta Katz (Charlotte, North Carolina); Thomas Kirsch (Konstanz); Tsitsi Masvaure (Massachusetts); Ruth Prince (Oslo); Petr Skalnik (Prague); and Eirik Saethre (Hawaii). The Niehaus family and my partner, Florence Bernault, have provided unfailing encouragement and support throughout the long process of research and writing.

Because my research has spanned many years, some of the material and thoughts contained in this book have already found their way into print. They appear in: 'Dr Wouter Basson, Americans and wild beasts: men's conspiracy theories of HIV/AIDS in the South African lowveld' (*Medical Anthropology* 24 (2): 177–206, 2005, with Gunvor Jonnson); 'Death before dying: understanding of AIDS stigma in the South African lowveld' (*Journal of Southern African Studies* 33 (4): 845–60, 2007); 'Leprosy of a deadlier kind: Christian conceptions of AIDS in the South African lowveld' (in F. Becker and W. Geissler (eds), *AIDS and Religious Practice in Africa*, Leiden: C. J. Brill, 2009); 'AIDS, speech and silence in South Africa' (*Anthropology Today* 29

(3): 8–12, 2013); 'Kuru, AIDS and witchcraft: reconfiguring culpability in Melanesia and in Africa' (*Social Analysis* 57 (3): 25–41, 2013); 'Treatment literacy, therapeutic efficacy and antiretroviral drugs: notes from Bushbuckridge, South Africa' (*Medical Anthropology* 33 (4): 351–66, 2013); and '"I don't want to hear": HIV, AIDS and the power of words in Bushbuckridge, South Africa' (in N. Beckman, A. Gusman, C. Shroff and R. van Dijk (eds), *Strings Attached: AIDS and the rise of transnational connections in Africa*, Oxford: Oxford University Press, 2014).

Isak Niehaus, Uxbridge, May 2018

I
Introduction

In 2001, the LoveLife AIDS awareness campaign established a Y-Centre at a trading centre near Impalahoek. LoveLife aimed to promote 'motivational optimism' and 'positive sexuality' as a lifestyle brand among local youth. The centre offered computer training, ballroom dancing, studio broadcasting and basketball. It also housed a 'wellness room', where youth received health-related counselling, and a 'chill room', where they read LoveLife literature. The Y-Centre attracted hundreds of young people.

Throughout my fieldwork, I nonetheless heard constant criticisms that LoveLife promoted urban American street styles. I was told that instructors taught attendants to sing the 'pizza' song: 'A Pizza Hut, a Pizza Hut, Kentucky Fried Chicken and a Pizza Hut, McDonald's, McDonald's'. During one promotional event, LoveLife parked a massive yacht on a trailer outside the centre to celebrate a voyage it had undertaken to Antarctica. The irony of the spectacle of a boat in the middle of a semi-arid environment did not go unnoticed by passers-by. Girls often played netball, a popular South African women's sport, on the basketball court (Wahlstrom 2002; Stadler 2011: 85–9). Residents also commented critically on a LoveLife poster that asked: 'If you aren't talking to your Child about Sex, Who Is? In vernacular kinship models, it is the obligation of the mother's brother (*malome*) and mother's younger sister (*mangwane*) – not of the mother and father – to speak to boys and girls about sexual matters.

The muted frictions arising from LoveLife's campaign demonstrate the salience of cultural miscommunication. Many villagers perceived earnest attempts to raise awareness about AIDS as alienating impositions. This was especially apparent when organisations such as LoveLife made dubious assumptions about the universal appropriateness of specific modes of entertainment, consumption, personal ambitions, games and ways of speech. Such initiatives seem to treat local meanings and practices as irrelevant, or as exotic exemplars of cultural difference that constitute barriers to HIV prevention and treatment. The latter stance is most apparent in the prejudicial views of polygamy, wife exchange, the levirate and dry sex as facilitating the spread of HIV in Africa (Gausset 2001).

One can rightly ask: where are the anthropologists? The marginalisation of anthropological expertise runs counter to the expectations of the enthusiastic founders the subdiscipline we now call medical anthropology. Physician-anthropologists such as Leslie (1976), Kleinman (1978) and Helman (1984) warned of the dangers of biomedical reductionism, which offered too limited a vision to grasp the complexities of health problems. Kleinman (1978) called on anthropologists to engage in comparative ethnographic research of medical systems as cultural systems and envisioned a key role for anthropologists as brokers within clinical practice and public health programmes. But the salience of bureaucratic logic and objectivity in international public health proved to be a formidable obstacle. Endeavours to measure morbidity and mortality rates have attracted far greater resources than attempts to understand 'lived experiences of sickness' (Kleinman 1995).

New orientations within anthropology itself have endangered the realisation of this original project. A focus on broad processes shaping our world, and on trans-local flows of pathogens, medical meanings and therapeutic resources (Petryna et al. 2006; Petryna 2009; Ong and Collier 2005), has eclipsed earlier concerns with the particularities of sickness and healing in specific settings. Influential proponents of world systems and globalisation theory go so far as to describe the fieldwork-based approach of Boas and Malinowski, which seeks to understand micro-level social relations, ritual and symbolism, as a 'wrong turn' in the history of anthropology (Wolf 1982; Singer 1989). More recently, a focus on the body and 'biopolitics' has also threatened to marginalise concerns with social and cultural specificities. Scholars contend that individuals increasingly perceive of themselves in somatic terms, and demand rights and resources based on their membership to universal biomedical categories (Petryna 2002; 2004). In the case of HIV/AIDS, influential analysts show how sick persons fashion new selves and novel modes of belonging through testing for HIV antibodies, participating in workshops, learning to speak publicly about AIDS, and using antiretroviral medication (Biehl 2007; Nguyen 2010). From this perspective, biomedical meanings and cosmopolitan lifestyles have, like steamrollers, obliterated existing social and symbolic forms. Biopolitical theorists do not suggest that cosmopolitan practices are uniquely appropriate, but they assert that these have attained problematic hegemony. From their vantage point, songs about McDonald's, aspirations about visiting Antarctica, basketball and free speech about sex have become integral features of the life worlds of local youth.

In this monograph, I seek to provide a detailed ethnographic account of how the HIV/AIDS pandemic unfolded in Impalahoek. In so doing, my aim is to formulate a more nuanced perspective on the way in which AIDS awareness and treatment programmes have intersected with existing social and symbolic forms; and to elucidate resultant 'frictions' in this regard (Tsing 2004). I contend that configurations that exist well beyond the clinic and other domains of professional healthcare – in the proverbial shadow of biomedicine – have profoundly shaped experiences of the pandemic. These include not only broader political and economic transitions – such as the end of apartheid, the entrenchment of African nationalism, and de-industrialisation – but also, and perhaps more relevant from an ethnographic perspective, meanings, practices and interpersonal relations that characterise everyday social interactions in the village setting.

Impalahoek is an appropriate site for such investigation. The village has one of the highest incidences of HIV infection worldwide. As insecurely employed labour migrants from a peripheral location, residents of Impalahoek have experienced the effects of broader political and economic fluctuations more acutely than securely employed workers from central locations. Yet, at the same time, the village is home to thriving folk traditions that are used to express difference, if not outright rejection, of cosmopolitan urban lifestyles (see Mitchell 2001: 12).

Empirically, I draw on the results of ongoing ethnographic research. Since 1990, I have visited Impalahoek for periods of at least four weeks each year, usually during the winter. Such episodic or multi-temporal fieldwork (Whyte 2013) has enabled me to observe the history of the pandemic over a 25-year period. I learned about daily life and events by doing participant observation and 'being around' political meetings, school staffrooms, hospitals, shops, football games, church services, rituals, divination sessions and funerals. I also conducted in-depth interviews specifically on the topic of HIV/AIDS with three different 'snowball' samples. Between 2002 and 2005, I recorded the sexual biographies of 27 men and documented their opinions about the origins and nature of HIV/AIDS. (Gunvor Jonnson interviewed 25 women to complement the material I collected.) I subsequently interviewed 21 persons who were diagnosed HIV-positive and used highly active antiretroviral therapy (HAART) about their experiences of sickness and therapy, and the heads of 22 households who were providing care for AIDS orphans. Although none of the samples are statistically representative,

I believe that they capture some of the diversities of experiences of HIV and AIDS among villagers in Impalahoek and also in the larger Bushbuckridge region.

All informants were previously known to my research assistants and had every right to refuse to participate. They were not offered any inducement, apart from the opportunity to contribute to the production of a history of the pandemic, which would be read by students and the members of future generations. Interviews were conducted in English, Northern Sotho and Tsonga and were recorded only in writing, because research participants feared that audiocassette recordings might compromise their anonymity. I relied on research assistants to translate difficult phrases in Northern Sotho and all narratives in Tsonga (a language I do not understand). We endeavoured to visit the research participants on separate occasions, to renew acquaintances and learn about how their lives had changed through time.

Research participants were generally confident and outspoken people who valued the opportunity to relay their own experiences and to speak out against the way in which the authorities had managed the pandemic. My status, not merely as a sympathetic outsider but also as a lone white person working with and among black people, constituted an important subtext to many interviews and conversations.[1] In Bushbuckridge, white people are most frequently businesspeople and doctors, and it is likely that some research participants might have associated me with hospital and clinic-based health workers. This perception was reinforced by the fact that I spoke openly about the potential benefits of antiretroviral therapy during interviews and might well have inhibited their criticisms of biomedical interventions. But these effects were mitigated by prior knowledge of my status as a student of history and of culture, and by the perception that white persons are generally opposed to many policies of South Africa's government.

Theoretically, my analysis of health-related interactions is inspired by Ortner's (1984) critique of a capitalist-centred world view, and by Sahlins' (1985; 1993) attempt to rethink colonial encounters in the Pacific islands. Ortner writes, very persuasively, that history is all too frequently treated 'as something that arrives like a ship, from outside the society in question (1984: 143). Whereas political economists tend to situate themselves on the ship, anthropologists have the unique capacity, developed largely through fieldwork, to 'take the perspective of folks on the shore' (ibid.: 143). For Sahlins, a central error of elite historiography is to presuppose a universal bourgeois subject and be unmindful of the culture of 'subalterns'. 'The agents of imperialism,' he writes, 'are not the exclusive players of the only game in town' (Sahlins 1993: 9). Sahlins contends that people understood and narrated events such as the arrival of Captain Cook in Hawai'i and the landing of British colonists in Karaka Bay, New Zealand, through established symbolic structures and storylines. They acted upon these through established forms of social organisation (Sahlins 1985; 1993).

Following Sahlins' and Ortner's lines of reasoning, I endeavour to show how residents of Impalahoek have understood AIDS-related sicknesses, and have engaged with biomedical interventions, through existing structures of meaning (pertaining to death, misfortune and dreams); and how they have acted upon these interventions through established modes of practice (allocating blame, speaking, seeking therapy, and taking care). Structures of meaning might well be more incoherent, permeable and amenable to contestation than Sahlins implies. There is also a danger that a critical focus on cultural idioms might ignore other forms of misrecognition, such as social class distinctions (Stadler and Hlongwa 2002; Hunter 2010). These lessons are well taken. We should use them as reasons to refine our attempts at understanding meaning and practice, rather than cast them out with the proverbial essentialist bathwater.

In the remainder of this chapter, I provide a critical overview of how what has come to be known as 'biopolitical' theory has shaped studies of HIV/AIDS, and why I believe such a theory has endangered an understanding of the social and cultural specificities of the pandemic. I then provide a brief history of Bushbuckridge, showing how popular discourses and sickness aetiologies have shaped experiences of HIV/AIDS. In the final part of this introduction, I outline the contours of my argument, as expressed in my organisation of the book.

Biopolitics and HIV/AIDS

Over the past two decades there has been a decisive shift in medical anthropology towards the somatic and to the body as 'subject of governance'. This interest was inspired by Foucault's (1973; 1977) and Agamben's (1998; 2005) observation that politics is increasingly situated at the level of biological life. Whereas earlier governments had invested in the power to 'make die and let live', Foucault contends that nineteenth-century European states used power to 'make life'. This project was marked by concerns with the welfare of populations and with the 'anatomo-politics' of individual bodies. By implementing measures to improve health, and by monitoring, regulating and disciplining the bodies of citizens, states began to intervene in the 'vital characteristics of human existence'. For Foucault, 'biopower' was exemplified by the development of scientific knowledge, and by the creation of institutions such as hospitals and asylums that implant modes of bodily conduct. 'Biopower' progressively extended beyond the state, to become dotted across the social landscape (Foucault 1980).

Agamben's (1998; 2005) analysis of sovereignty begins with a discussion of the *homo sacer*. This obscure category in Roman law denoted a person whose crimes disqualified him or her from being a sacrificial victim, but whom anyone could kill with impunity. For Agamben, this legal category continued to be a hidden aspect of power, because the right to take life remained intrinsic to sovereignty. This is evident in the capacity of states to enforce 'states of exception' in which they suspend the rule of law in the name of 'self-defence'. The threat of confining persons to zones of torture and death backs up the commands of government and extends to experts such as jurists and doctors who exercise authority over the vital existence of humans.

Rose (2001; 2006) and Rabinow and Rose (2006) develop these insights. They observe that contemporary developments in genetics, the neuro-sciences and medical technology have led to a resurgence of biological accounts of human capacities. In the emerging 'biopolitics', power relations attain a 'pastoral appearance'. States and private corporations create the conditions for – and enhance the obligations of – individuals to manage their own health.[2] These agents embrace statistical reasoning and recommend preventative interventions to reduce risks. Such interventions to protect 'bare life' and restrict 'defective' biological propensities expand and refine strategies of control. In this process, the body is transformed into a site for working on and modifying the self. Individuals increasingly perceive the self in terms of the functioning of genes and molecules and become active participants in the 'will to health' (Rose 2001: 7). They see biology as improvable, invest in economies of hope, and change their life course through acts of choice.

According to Rose and Novas (2005) and Rabinow and Rose (2006), these developments pave the way for the emergence of new forms of citizenship and sociality. Biomedical technologies increasingly yield categories of social import. These categories have come to underpin the way in which authorities 'make up citizens' (Rose and Novas 2005: 440), and also the manner in which people claim entitlement to participate in political affairs: for example, people with neurofibromatosis meet to share experiences and lobby for resources. In certain situations, activism becomes the norm and citizens become 'moral pioneers' who shape new ways of understanding and acting upon themselves (ibid.: 451).

In a detailed study, Petryna (2002; 2004) shows how the Chernobyl nuclear disaster of 1986 created a new political field in the Ukraine, in which forms of the state and citizenship were remade. Persons who had been exposed to radiation effects claimed rights to health services and support in the name of their damaged bodies. Through such activism, they learned to use biological rationalities to negotiate terms of social and economic inclusion. The Chernobyl disaster also created an economy of medical suffering and radiation expertise, and generated legal criteria for acknowledging injury and compensation.

The constellation of AIDS-related diseases provides an interesting test case for biopolitical theory. The pandemic emerged precisely at the same time as accelerated developments occurred in the biological sciences and technologies. Yet 95 per cent of HIV infections occur in the global South, where severe resource shortages undermine the hegemony of biomedicine. The first ethnographic studies focused on how sexual networks and relations facilitated the spread of HIV (Setel 1999; Boyce 2007; Gutmann 2007; Thornton 2008) and on how affected communities made sense of the disease and coped with sickness and death (Pigg 2001; Fordham 2004; Butt 2005; Butt and Eves 2008). These studies were sensitive to the specificities of local settings and paved the way for inter-contextual understanding. But with the introduction of antiretroviral treatment, attention shifted to global assemblages of biomedical resources, finance and knowledge; transnational health interventions; and novel forms of biopolitical belonging and activism.

Biehl's and Nguyen's work most clearly exemplifies this approach. Biehl (2004) suggests that Brazilian initiatives challenge the assumption that low-income countries cannot intervene in the pandemic's course. In Brazil, the pandemic accentuated the integration of biotechnology into public policy. In 1992, the state invested $250 million on AIDS programmes, focusing on condom distribution, testing for HIV antibodies, and behaviour change. By 1998, it was providing free antiretroviral drugs to 58,000 patients, at an annual cost of $300 million. The Brazilian government acted in concert with grassroots movements and gay rights activists, who struggled to secure treatment as a right of citizenship. President Cardoza used the pandemic as leverage to circumvent patent protection for pharmaceuticals and facilitate the local production of generics. The pandemic also allowed for the making of novel forms of inclusion and exclusion. Testing and risk assessments brought individuals under systemic monitoring and ingrained health-based concepts of citizenship (ibid.: 109). But homeless persons, drug users and commercial sex workers with AIDS remained invisible to the state, and could access pharmaceuticals only through community-run houses of support.

Nguyen (2010) argues that, in West Africa, where he worked as an HIV clinician, the scarcity of clinical resources did not diminish the power of biomedicine. Instead, the biomedical fraternity came to exercise a kind of 'therapeutic sovereignty'. By allocating scarce therapeutic resources, physicians engaged in a form of triage, deciding who would live and who would die.[3] The erosion of state power through structural adjustment and multiparty politics enhanced the prominence of physicians. Moreover, Nguyen contends that HIV-infected persons learned to fashion the self in relation to existing moral codes in order to access therapy. Testing for HIV antibodies, attending workshops and talking publicly about one's illness were prerequisites for obtaining antiretroviral drugs. He sketches vivid portraits of how AIDS awareness used testimonials to construct social networks and claim 'therapeutic citizenship' on the basis of a shared biomedical condition. Nguyen also shows how 'confessional technologies' are transported from Brussels to Washington to Abidjan, and how entrepreneurs use their transnational networks as conduits for access to drugs and jobs.

The South African situation, where protracted political struggles preceded the distribution of HAART, poses different analytical challenges. Here, President Thabo Mbeki explicitly resisted calls by health activists to provide the drugs AZT and nevirapine to pregnant women infected with HIV.[4] Instead, Mbeki supported the view of dissident scientists that people diagnosed as living with AIDS suffered from poverty-related diseases, and that pharmaceutical corporations merely promoted antiretroviral drugs (ARVs) because they had vested financial interest in their use. In 2003, the Treatment Action Campaign (TAC) successfully filed a case in the High Court, forcing the South African government to make ARVs available through public healthcare facilities, in order to satisfy patients' constitutional right to life. Subsequently, the national health department – supported by the Global Fund to Fight AIDS, Tuberculosis and Malaria, and the United States President's Emergency Plan for AIDS Relief (PEPFAR) – implemented a national roll-out of HAART. But the South African government consistently failed to meet its own targets in supplying antiretroviral drugs,[5] and repeatedly commented on their toxic side effects.

South African academics were generally critical of President Mbeki's policies, and often conceptualised the struggle for affordable medication as a contest between 'science' and 'ignorance' (Mbali 2004; Geffin 2005; Leclerc-Madlala 2005; Natrass 2007; 2012). The most influential studies framed these struggles as biopolitical ones. Fassin (2007) appears to be more sympathetic to President Mbeki and discusses the broader context of his policies. His central thesis is that the bodies of persons suffering from AIDS-related diseases bore testimony to a long history of racism, political repression and economic inequality. Fassin's analysis is overtly critical of 'culturalist' readings of HIV/AIDS. Claire Laurier Decoteau (2013) relates President Mbeki's controversial stance to 'neoliberal' economic restructuring, and his desire to see South Africa prosper on international markets, without being dependent on Western nations. Such restructuring is evident in the government's reliance on 'the community' to undertake responsibility for home-based care. She nonetheless argues that these policies amounted to a form of 'thanato-politics', in which the state assumed sovereign power to disallow life.

Robins (2004; 2006) discusses activism for affordable medication as a quest for 'biological citizenship'. He contends that TAC activists used new languages to forge transnational alliances and to produce empowered and responsible citizens who were aware of their rights and entitlements, and were able to adhere effectively to treatment regimes. Robins shows how programmes launched by the TAC and by MSF (Médecins Sans Frontières) to supply free HAART in Cape Town radically transformed the subjectivities of persons living with AIDS. Patients using HAART provided testimonies that recount a journey from 'bare life' – of sickness and isolation – to a 'new life' – of health and acceptance. They literally transformed the stigma of HIV/AIDS into a 'badge of pride', displayed on T-shirts at workshops, funerals and demonstrations (Robins 2006: 314). Likewise, Fassin and colleagues show how persons living with AIDS in Johannesburg used biographical narratives to overcome pathos, access social grants, and secure employment as educators within non-government organisations (NGOs) operating in the domain of AIDS (Fassin et al. 2008: 234).

From biopolitical theory to social specificity

Biopolitical theory confers valuable insights and perspectives. But it also has definite weaknesses, limitations and analytical blind spots, which preclude a nuanced understanding of the full complexity of responses to the HIV/AIDS pandemic in marginal places such as Impalahoek.

These include the inappropriate conception of agency, and a narrow analytical focus on biomedical understandings and therapies. For Sahlins (2004), Foucauldian theories about the transmission of social order to individual bodies threaten to dissolve persons into victims of the hegemonic order. By equating social forms with specific subject positions, these theories ignore the unique biographies of persons. Sahlins quotes Sartre: 'Valéry is a petit bourgeois individual – not every petit bourgeois individual is Valéry' (Sartre 1960: 55–6). In anthropological terms, biopolitical theory privileges the universal and endangers an understanding of the specificities, not only of individuals but also of the social and cultural contexts that shape their lives.

With rare exceptions, such as Petryna's work on the Ukraine, studies of biopolitics are imprecise about their units of observation and analysis. This has created the impression of an ethnocentric assumption that experiences in wealthier Northern countries are normative for the globe. Biopolitical theory also privileges concerns with events in biomedical and clinical domains over those in domestic ones. Rose and Novas recognise that 'vectors from below introduce doubt and controversy' (2005: 447), and that the capacity of genetics to define new forms of citizenship varies, according to the availability of resources and concepts of personhood. 'Certain forms of biosociality,' they write, 'have no presence in whole geographical regions' (ibid.: 448). But what, precisely, are these vectors from below? And, what happens in zones beyond the biopolitical?

These questions are particularly apposite in continents such as Africa, where thriving traditions of medical pluralism attest to the relevance of ideas about health, beyond the biomedical (Olsen and Sargent 2017). Prince writes that, throughout Africa, biomedicine coexists 'with other epistemologies and practices that locate health and therapy in arenas beyond the biological body, outside the clinic and the hospital and among non-biomedical authorities' (2013: 6).

A more appropriate theoretical vantage point for this monograph is a body of works that examine how people in specific African social settings deal with HIV/AIDS (Geissler and Becker 2009; Geissler and Prince 2012; Dilger and Luig 2010; Marsland and Prince 2012; Reynolds Whyte 2014). These authors do not assume the unproblematic hegemony of biomedical paradigms, but pay special attention to life worlds beyond the clinic. Although they are frequently based on more in-depth fieldwork than studies rooted in biopolitical theory, they have, perhaps for reasons of fashion, attracted less notice.

A prominent example is the 'polygraph' by Reynolds Whyte and her Danish and Ugandan colleagues (2014), which documents the experiences of the first generation of Ugandans on HAART. Based on extensive research within local village settings, the authors follow the concerns of their interlocutors rather than those of global health actors, and focus on everyday forms of interaction, beyond the purview of health policymakers.

The authors single out issues pertaining to generation, sociality and 'second chances' for discussion. They describe their interlocutors as a 'bio-generation' for whom experiences with AIDS and HAART were iconic in their acquisition of modes of behaviour, feeling and thought. But their interlocutors also came of age during a period of nation building after civil war by President Museveni, and of a resurgence of Pentecostal churches. In Uganda, AIDS awareness programmes and Christian revivalism affected each other in several ways. This is evident in the advocacy of chastity, monogamy and faithfulness, and in the conjunction of physical and spiritual salvation.

Reynolds Whyte argues that in Uganda the concept of 'clientship', based on personal relations of dependence, captures the use of therapeutic services better than 'citizenship', based on the therapeutic rights of individuals vis-à-vis the same polity (2014: 17). She also observes that participation in networks of kinship counterbalances the formation of bio-sociality. 'Events and representations were mediated by the social relations in which the actors were already embedded, including those with parents and children' (ibid.: 17). This implies a paradoxical generational consciousness. On the one hand, public testimonials were decisive to obtaining therapy; on the other, silence was necessary to avoid the discrediting effects of AIDS stigma among colleagues, kin and neighbours.[6]

HAART enabled some members of this generation to make a decisive break with the past, and gave them an opportunity to be 'born again' and lead a better, more positive life. It provided others with a stay of execution, and a chance to resume their lives and return to the everyday. They viewed the ability to live an ordinary life, after confronting life-threatening sickness, as an achievement

(Reynolds White 2014: 20). Meinert observes that, for persons on HAART, the desire to participate in the economy and family, and to engage in sex and reproduction, were often more sustained concerns than becoming 'citizens' in a pharmaceutical sense (2014: 136).

Like Biehl and Nguyen, Reynolds Whyte et al. (2014) write a great deal more about the experiences of sick people using HAART than about those who do not. But they adopt a more open-ended approach that is attentive to the way in which religion, ideology and kinship permeate biomedical concerns. They do not treat biological citizenship as stable, but as perennially contingent and insecure (see Hull 2017).

A host of ethnographic studies on HIV/AIDS in South Africa contest key assumptions in biopolitical theory concerning the flow of biomedical meanings and treatments. These show how people in different township and village settings reject, contest or bypass the messages propagated by AIDS awareness initiatives. Ashforth (2002) observes that residents of Soweto interpreted the symptoms of AIDS as an effect of a slow poison, called *isidliso*, inflicted by witches. The poison allegedly came in the form of a small creature that gradually devoured and slowly consumed the victims' bodies from the inside.

According to Stadler (2011) and McNeill (2009), the model of 'biological citizens' who deploy confessional technologies find little resonance in the former Gazankulu and Venda Bantustans. Here, in Stadler's (2011) words, village residents 'conceal suffering' and treat HIV/AIDS as a 'shared secret'. Despite being knowledgeable about biomedical constructions, people refrained from speaking about HIV/AIDS at public events. To do so would be to embarrass and shame. Instead, they articulated AIDS through gossip and rumour that resisted dominant epidemiological explanations (Stadler 2003b). Local narratives imposed moral readings on behaviour and referred to unscrupulous sexual conduct by young adults, miracle cures by diviners, doctors injecting patients with HIV-contaminated blood, and government lacing condoms with the 'AIDS worms' (McNeill 2009).

Strategies for prevention and treatment have also been unpredictable. Leclerc-Madlala (2001) and Scorgie (2002) discerned a resurgence of neo-traditional virginity-testing ceremonies in Zululand, in which senior women examine girls to ensure the maintenance of feminine purity. Also, the public sector roll-out of HAART has not imposed biomedical hegemony. Decoteau (2013) observes that few residents of the informal settlements around Johannesburg endorsed the ideology of 'scientific salvation' propagated by the TAC.[7] In addition to using HAART, sick residents consulted diviners, invoked the ancestors, used herbs, and underwent Christian cleansing rituals. They remained mindful of the limits of biomedicine and perceived connections between bodies and broader social and spiritual networks. In Bushbuckridge, men receiving HAART have been extremely reluctant to embrace 'HIV-positive identities'. Mfecane's (2011) male research participants gained the knowledge and skills necessary for adherence but saw treatment regimens as constraining. They resisted the 'sick' role, which deprived them of autonomy; they continued to see proscribed behaviour such as drinking beer as essential to masculine sociability; and they still used herbs to cleanse themselves from dirt.

These discordant examples reveal various muted forms of contestation and hidden forms of 'resistance' (Scott 1990) to the imposition of biomedical understandings of HIV/AIDS and its treatment in South Africa. But more than this, the examples point to the limitations of biomedical paradigms in dealing with specificity and difference. In spatial terms, global flows do not have homogenising outcomes, and they forge not only connections but also disconnections (Ferguson 1999; Cooper 2001). In temporal terms, the imposition of biomedical treatment does not imply a clean break with the past. We might well be wiser to assume the existence of both continuities and discontinuities and seek to understand how new therapeutic practices interact with and overlay existing meanings and social relations.

To me, Reynolds Whyte's open-ended approach offers a more appropriate point of departure for understanding the complexities of HIV/AIDS in Impalahoek. In this book, I also seek to build on the insights of studies on South Africa. Rather than focus on the flow of biomedical taxonomies and responses to them, I acknowledge a situation of medical pluralism. Here, Bourdieu's (1991) notion of a changing social field in which different actors compete to accumulate symbolic and social capital comes to mind. This open-ended perspective is also evident in Foucault's (1980) recognition that power is not brought to bear on sexual conduct through a unitary scientific discourse, but through multiple dispersed and competing discursive frameworks. This seems to be as pertinent to sickness and healing as it is to sexuality.

Sickness and AIDS: a brief history of Bushbuckridge

In the brief history below, I endeavour to demonstrate how pluralism characterised ways of understanding and dealing with sickness and misfortune in Bushbuckridge, and how these were intertwined with changing political, economic and social contexts. While the AIDS pandemic did generate a proliferation of biomedical discourses, people's experiences of them were deeply embedded in epistemologies and practices that existed beyond clinics, hospitals and public health forums.

The current population of Bushbuckridge are descendants of diverse Northern Sotho (Bakone, Baroka and Pulana) and Tsonga-speaking groups (Banwalungu, Hlanganu and Nxumalo) who settled beneath the Moholoholo mountains from the mid-nineteenth century onwards. During the late 1880s, encroachment by white settlers altered their conditions of life. President Kruger's government surveyed and sold large tracts of land to speculators and granted Afrikaner men 'occupation farms' in exchange for 'military service' (Harries 1989: 91). The new landlords initially compelled Africans resident on their land to pay rent in cash and kind. But a 'labour tenancy' system gradually emerged, under the terms of which African men worked for the white landlord over a period of three months each year, without remuneration. For the remainder of the year, they and other household members cultivated their own fields, tended their own cattle, or migrated to work in the South African goldmines (ibid.: 93–4).

The Native Land Act of 1913 scheduled many farms, including in Impalahoek, for exclusive African occupation. Here, it left intact a system of 'rent-tenancy', whereby residents of the farms paid taxes to landholding companies for residential, cultivation and stock-keeping rights. The settlement pattern was one of scattered hamlets (*metse*) that comprised the homesteads, fields, gardens and ancestral graves of co-resident agnatic clusters. Until the early 1930s, fields were still basically as large as a hamlet could cultivate and no stock limitations were imposed. In a good year, the wealthiest hamlets harvested up to 90 bags of maize plus 30 bags of sorghum and kept herds of more than 150 cattle. They paid rent by selling produce and stock to traders. Men also worked intermittently in forestry plantations or in the Pilgrim's Rest goldmines to obtain cash for clothes and other commodities.

Since the 1930s, thousands of displaced households moved onto company farms, such as Impalahoek. This was due to the creation of the Kruger National Park towards the east, the afforestation of

Mount Moholoholo in the west, and the expulsion of former labour tenants from the white-owned farms, where production operations were increasingly mechanised. This influx of people placed increased strain on rural resources, leading to soil erosion and greater vulnerability to drought. Under these conditions, more men signed up to longer migrant labour contracts and also started to work further afield, such as in the Witwatersrand, where they could earn higher wages.

In 1948, the year when apartheid became official government policy, the South African Native Trust purchased all company farms to create the Bushbuckridge Native Reserve (Niehaus et al. 2001: 21). This facilitated an influx of even more African households into the area (Harries 1989: 104). Having failed to acquire more land, the Native Affairs Department altered the use of land in Bushbuckridge. Field officers demarcated clearly defined residential, arable and grazing areas in the reserve. Whereas households had previously had an average of 2.5 hectares of land, they were now allocated only 0.8 hectares for agriculture.[8] Few households could produce more than six bags of maize on their reduced fields. In addition, they suffered great losses when a devastating epizootic outbreak decimated their cattle herds in 1951.

Within the context of diminishing rural resources, local cosmologies linked misfortune and sickness to the workings of coexisting metaphysical powers inhering in spiritual agencies, persons, and nature. A widely held belief was that cognatic ancestors (*badimo*), whose blood (*madi*) was present in the bodies of their descendants and whose breath (*moya*) continued to hover around their homestead, displayed continued parental concern over the living. To ensure their protective support, villagers acquired items such as old coins or walking sticks and built small circular homes (*ndumba*) for their ancestors. In times of distress, households invoked the ancestors, or sacrificed cows by their gravesides, to secure their assistance.

The earliest diviner-healers (*dingaka*) were men who were favoured by their ancestors and who acquired their skills through extended periods of apprenticeship. Diviners discovered the source of distress by casting divination lots, and treated sickness by prescribing herbs. However, the settlement of Shangaans in Bushbuckridge saw the advent of more powerful diviner-healers (*inyanga*). The first were a woman, Nkomo We Lwandle ('Cow of the Ocean'), and a man, Dunga Manzi ('Stirring Water'), who had reportedly been trained by a mysterious water serpent (*nzunzu*).[9] These Shangaan diviners and their apprentices interpreted persistent ailments as signs that foreign spirits troubled their clients. These spirits included the Malopo (who were Sotho), the Ngoni (who were Shangaan, Zulu and Swazi), and the fierce Ndzau (from Musapa in Mozambique). During a ritual, which included drumming, instructors exhorted the spirits to speak through the mouth of the afflicted person and state their demands. Once appeased, the spirits gradually bestowed the powers of divination, foresight and healing upon their mediums. The Malopo specialised in healing venereal diseases and sick children; the Ngoni in treating paralysis and skin diseases; and the Ndzau in detecting witchcraft.

Witchcraft beliefs located sickness in the nexus of interpersonal relationships. The term 'witch' (*moloi*; plural: *baloi*) denotes a person who inherited malevolent capacities from their mother or purchased harmful substances and skills from others. Witches allegedly used poisons (*tshefu*), such as the notorious crocodile brain. They also manufactured potions (*dihlare*) from organic materials – roots, barks, animal fats and even substances from the human body. When placed on footpaths, such potions caused paralysis of the legs; when placed in the forest, they caused winds to drive away dark, rain-bearing clouds. In addition, witches by birth sent out familiars (*dithuri*) – usually snakes, owls, hyenas, baboons, cats and even lions – to attack their victims at night. The aim of witchcraft was the cannibalistic consumption of the victim's flesh. But witches could also change their victims into nocturnal servants (*ditlotlwane*; translated to me as zombies). Until the 1960s, most witchcraft accusations occurred between neighbours and relatives by marriage, and they were an index of tensions over unequal harvests and troubled relations between mothers and daughters-in-law (Niehaus et al. 2001: 133–9).

The transgression of taboos (*dilla*) constituted an additional source of danger. The observance of these showed respect for nature. For example, it was taboo to plant bean or pumpkin in summer, fell certain trees, and cut reeds from the time of sowing until harvesting. Such deeds invited winds and drought. Other taboos pertained to the maintenance of rank and to the avoidance of contact with the polluting heat (*fiša*) of corpses, pregnant women and women who had recently aborted. Senior houses were obliged to taste the crops of the new season before junior houses, and sons were expected to marry in sequence of age. To avert contamination by death, bereaved families observed a week-long period of mourning, during which they abstained from sexual intercourse, ceased working in the fields, and refrained from touching young children. Widows, who had the most intimate contact with the deceased, observed a year-long period of mourning. Transgressions of these taboos generated different afflictions. Children who met an adult in a state of heat contracted *makgoma*, which was marked by convulsions and shortness of breath. Transgressions of funeral taboos brought about *mafulara*, the symptoms of which were severe chest pains and profuse coughing. Sexual intercourse with women who had recently been widowed or aborted generated *lešiši*, a potentially fatal condition characterised by internal bleeding.

Christian missions and schools, which provided an alternative religious framework, constructed the first schools and clinical facilities in Bushbuckridge. In 1936, the American Nazarene Church and International Holiness Mission built the Ethel Lucas Memorial Hospital east of Impalahoek. By 1948, the hospital had 66 beds and a permanent medical practitioner, and treated about 5,000 patients per annum (Nkuna 1986: 151). Women participated most eagerly in the activities of the missions, through which they gained entry to the teaching and nursing professions (ibid.: 181; Hull 2017: 87–120).

Interventions by the apartheid government further transformed social and economic life in Bushbuckridge. During 1959, Bantu authorities were established in Bushbuckridge, and chiefs became accountable to white Bantu affairs commissioners. The next year, officials of the Bantu Trust implemented a comprehensive 'agricultural betterment' scheme to ease pressure on rural resources. The officials re-divided all land into new residential settlements, arable fields and grazing camps. Given the diminutive size of these residential stands, large agnatic clusters were fragmented into smaller households. Very few households secured access to arable fields, and none were permitted to keep more than ten head of cattle (Niehaus et al. 2001: 29–30). Proletarianisation was now complete, and labour migration became a masculine career. During 1962, in accordance with broader apartheid policies, the government divided the entire Native Reserve along ethnic lines. The eastern side, designated as Mhala, became part of the Shangaan Bantustan, Gazankulu, in 1969; the western side, in which Impalahoek was situated, was called Mapulaneng and incorporated into the Northern Sotho Bantustan of Lebowa in 1973.

Subtle changes also occurred in the ecology of beliefs pertaining to misfortune and sickness. The 1960s saw a phenomenal growth of Zionist and Apostolic churches, their influence rapidly eclipsing that of the older Christian missions (Niehaus et al. 2001: 32). The ZCC (Zion Christian Church) soon became the largest church in Impalahoek.[10] Formed in 1924 by Bishop Engenas Lekganyane, the ZCC comprised thousands of dispersed rural congregations throughout Southern Africa. Its structure resembled that of chiefly authority, descending from an archbishop to ministers (*baruti*), prophets, secretaries and treasurers. Each Easter, buses carried hundreds of thousands of worshippers to the church's headquarters at Moria, near Polokwane, where the archbishop would address the uniformed multitudes over electronic sound systems. Smaller Apostolic congregations, led by bishops and prophets who claimed guidance from the Holy Spirit, and Pentecostal churches also secured footholds in Impalahoek.

These churches constituted a broader domain of sociality than the household, compensating for the demise of large agnatic clusters. They also provided a novel framework for health maintenance and healing. The attraction of Zionist and Apostolic churches stemmed from their 'this world' emphasis on harnessing the divine power of the Holy Spirit to reconstruct people's immediate life worlds (Comaroff 1985: 240). This orientation is apparent in the practices of river baptism, purification, prohibitions on drinking and smoking, uniformed dancing and night communions. The practices of Apostolic healers, who treated patients at home, resembled those of diviners. They would cast a multicoloured string cord to the ground and claim that, through its position, the Holy Spirit revealed aspects of their patients' conditions to them. The healers then used prayer and remedies prescribed by the Holy Spirit (*ditaelo*) to effect healing.

The churches recast existing metaphysical powers in a dualistic framework of good and evil. Christians emphasised the benevolence of cognatic ancestors, whom they believed acted in a subsidiary capacity to the Holy Spirit. Church leaders mentioned God's commandment that one should honour and obey one's parents. But through the churches Christians devised alternative ways of placating the ancestors: instead of conducting blood sacrifice, ministers prayed that descendants might be reconciled with their deceased relatives. Among Christians, attention shifted from traditional taboos to the 'laws of churches', such as the Ten Commandments and the dietary prohibitions of Leviticus. Because agriculture was no longer the source of people's livelihood, actions that caused drought (such as cutting reeds in the wrong season) inspired less fear. But church members still upheld older taboos pertaining to seniority, birth, sex and death. Local congregations required that mothers be secluded with their newborn infants for a period of up to two months, supervised funerals, and required widows to wear the mourning attire of the church. At home, senior daughters still sowed before junior ones, and children tasted the new crops in sequence of age. Households also ensured that children did not meet people in states of heat (*fiša*). The relations between the churches and healer-diviners, who served as mediums for foreign spirits, were generally tense. Ministers sometimes understood these spirits to be demons. But diviners themselves contested this representation and insisted that the spirits could be helpful. One episode was widely discussed. In 1975, ministers of the Nazarene Revival Crusade called two women diviners servants of Satan and commanded them to burn their regalia. After this, both became seriously ill. Only after they left the church and rededicated themselves to the spirits did the women regain their health.

Witchcraft accusations escalated under the dual impact of villagisation, which brought greater distrust between neighbours, and the Manichean world view propagated by the churches. Villagers feared that migrants brought new and ever more dangerous witch familiars, such as the ape-like *tokolotši* and snake-like *mamlambo*, from urban markets into Bushbuckridge. Witches allegedly sent the *tokolotši*, which had pronounced sexual features, to rape desirable women and men in their neighbourhoods, and commanded the *mamlambo* to bring them wealth. But, in return for money, the snake would demand the blood of its keeper's kin (Niehaus 1995). Despite escalating fears of bewitchment, Bantu affairs commissioners strictly upheld the Suppression of Witchcraft Act (No. 3) of 1957, which explicitly prohibited diviners from pointing out witches, and chiefs from interfering in witchcraft accusations.[11] In this context, Zionist and Apostolic healers assumed greater responsibility for managing anxieties about witchcraft. For them, unlike earlier missionaries, witches constituted a more immediate source of evil than Satan (Kiernan 1997). But their response was always defensive. Christian healers did not confront alleged witches but used prescriptions from the Holy Spirit to protect church members against witchcraft and to heal witchcraft-related diseases.

Biomedicine gradually lost its Christian moorings. In 1973, administration of the Ethel Lucas Memorial Hospital passed from mission churches to the Gazankulu Department of Health. This department renamed the hospital Tintswalo ('mercy' in Tsonga) and largely appointed Shangaans to new positions. Northern Sotho speakers did not feel particularly welcome, especially at the time of land disputes between Gazankulu and Lebowa. To avoid discrimination, some preferred to attend Lebowa's Masana Hospital, located 35 kilometres further away. Tintswalo increasingly dealt with diseases such as tuberculosis that were associated with poverty and labour

migration (De Beer 1984). Teachers and civil servants of the Bantustans, whose remuneration packages included medical insurance,
started consulting private doctors, whom they believed provided a
better service.

The anti-apartheid struggle brought a proliferation of political discourses to Bushbuckridge. From 1986, male youths called
comrades, who allied themselves with national liberation movements,
aggressively confronted all institutions they associated with the
apartheid system. Organising from local schools, comrades enforced
a series of boycotts of educational institutions, white-owned supermarkets, and government taxes. They also dedicated themselves to
the complete eradication of evil. Comrades called a series of meetings at which they asked adult men to name suspected witches. They
then formed disciplinary squads to punish the accused. Between
April and May 1986, the comrades burned hundreds of homes and
attacked at least 150 suspected witches (SAIRR 1988: 907).

The ANC (African National Congress) was unbanned in February
1990. The organisation immediately established new branches in
Bushbuckridge, and rapidly won over not only the youth but also
their former enemies, such as Bantustan leaders, chiefs, businessmen
and school principals. In 1994, the ANC secured a dramatic victory
during South Africa's first democratic elections – claiming 92 per
cent of all votes cast in Limpopo Province. Through participating
in these elections, villagers sought to achieve political representation in national centres of power and saw African nationalism as an
eminently suitable vehicle for this purpose.

South Africa's new government disestablished all Bantustan
structures. Impalahoek now came to be administered by the newly
constituted Bushbuckridge municipality and, eventually, also by
Mumpalanga Province.[12] The first two decades of democratic rule
brought increased differentiation and some out-migration. The
village population, still numbering more than 20,000 people, became
increasingly heterogeneous. A new, albeit small, elite emerged,
comprising well-paid civil servants and business people who secured
lucrative service provision tenders from government. Members
of this class have either moved to townships with proper urban
infrastructure, such as Dwarsloop, or have constructed large, ostentatious homes surrounded by high security walls. Some white-collar
workers, such as salespersons, and skilled manual labourers, such
as truck drivers, immigrated to the cities of Gauteng and had only
tenuous connections with Impalahoek. Other professionals, such as
teachers and police officers, remained, sometimes living in the same

households as less fortunate kin. Ordinary households frequently complained of deteriorating economic conditions (Niehaus 2005). The downsizing of factories and the closure of mines in South Africa's industrial centres meant drastic job losses, particularly among men. Unemployment in Impalahoek was considerably higher than the national average of 27 per cent (Peyper 2017), and workers such as taxi drivers, security guards and seasonal farm labourers were relatively poorly remunerated and lacked job security. Numerous households were dependent for their livelihood on social security payments, such as old age and disability pensions, and child maintenance and foster grants.[13]

Despite direct experiences of broader political and economic transformations sweeping through the African subcontinent in recent years, Impalahoek still had a distinctively rural appearance. Village roads were of gravel and sand, and were poorly maintained. There was no rubbish removal system, and homes were more likely to have fridges and television sets than onsite water and sewerage. Goats commonly grazed on unoccupied residential stands, and in each village section cattle owners collectively hired the services of a herder to take their stock to grazing camps during the day. Immigrants from Mozambique and Zimbabwe had a visible presence, and there were now also Ethiopian, Somali, Pakistani and Chinese immigrants, who ran small trading enterprises. Although the ZCC remained dominant, some youth now attended new Pentecostal-type churches, sporting names such Living Purpose Ministry, Hope Fellowship and Waters of Life. There was also an emerging consumer culture, centred on a shopping mall on the eastern outskirts of Impalahoek, which hosted two large supermarkets, fast-food outlets, and several furniture and clothing stores. Young adults frequently purchased goods on credit, or took out high-interest loans, resulting in crippling debts.

Politically, there has been growing discontent about the lack of progress in service delivery, escalating crime, and the different forms of corruption that beset Jacob Zuma's presidency. Villagers became more inclined to vote for opposition parties, and, since 2012, candidates of the Bushbuckridge Residents Association (BRA) have defeated those of the ANC in municipal council elections.

The first AIDS-related deaths in Impalahoek occurred during the early 1990s. Comprehensive verbal autopsy surveys conducted annually by epidemiologists on common signs and symptoms of death in Agincourt, another village of Bushbuckridge, aptly demonstrate how HIV and AIDS progressively assumed pandemic proportions.[14] Until 1995, infectious diseases and malnutrition were the predominant causes of death among children, accidents and violence were the main causes among adolescents and young adults, and cardiovascular diseases among the middle-aged and elderly. But between 1995 and 2002, AIDS was the most frequent cause of death in all age groups (Tollman et al. 1999). Between 1992 and 2005, life expectancy in Agincourt decreased by 14 years for women and by 12 years for men (Kahn et al. 2007).

The first initiatives to stem the spread of HIV emanated from NGOs and focused on the awareness and prevention of AIDS. In 1992, the Health Systems Development Unit at Tintswalo hospital launched a sexual health programme. Three staff members gave talks on sexual hygiene to constituencies such as the police, clergy, headmen and diviners, and to teachers and learners in schools. The unit also established sexual health clinics, and trained youth as peer educators. At the same time, unpaid volunteers of the Bushbuckridge Health and Social Service Consortium (BHSSC) provided information and support to people living with AIDS, and the Acornhoek Reproductive Health Youth Groups Project organised an educational outreach programme in six local schools. In 2000, an ostentatious LoveLife youth centre was built. The centre employed five permanent staff members, ten 'groundbreakers' (who introduce LoveLife to the public), and 30 unpaid volunteers. They marketed safe sex as part of a 'lifestyle brand', focused on global youth culture (Wahlstrom 2002; Stadler and Hlongwa 2002).

Whereas a large amount of publicity surrounded safe sex, the victims of AIDS-related diseases were shielded from public view and compelled to die slowly at home. A network of three hospitals and six clinics screened pregnant women for seroprevalence and administered free tests for HIV antibodies on request, but they treated only the symptoms of AIDS. In addition, the Rixile ('Rising Sun' in Tsonga) Wellness Clinic, established by the Witwatersrand University's School of Public Health at Tintswalo hospital, supported people with AIDS and helped them apply for disability grants.

Only during 2003, following approval from government, did private doctors and Masana Hospital begin to supply free antiretroviral medication to patients whose CD4 count tested below 200[15] and who had demonstrated psychosocial preparedness to take up therapy. In 2005, Rixile clinic began to roll out HAART and provide extensive treatment literacy training.[16] By October that year, some 1,500 people regularly attended the clinic, and by 2008 this number had grown to 6,000. HAART could potentially transform AIDS from a terminal condition into a chronic, manageable sickness, and literally reclaim life from death. Within months, the weight of one patient attending Rixile increased from 20 kilograms to 70 kilograms. Clinical evidence has shown reasonable success. Researchers monitored 1,353 patients who were initiated on HAART at Rixile over a 24-month period. Despite late presentation, 84 per cent (1,131) were retained on treatment, 9 per cent (124) had died, 5 per cent (63) had been transferred out, and 3 per cent (35) could not be traced (MacPherson et al. 2008: 590).

Medical infrastructure, outside the clinic, remained rudimentary. By 2008, Rixile's services still reached only 20 per cent of those in its catchment area (MacPherson et al. 2008: 592). Low government spending on health, and the expansion of the global market in medical skills, also generated inefficiencies and a severe shortage in medical personnel (Hull 2017: 86–8). In 2010, Tintswalo hospital was a 423-bed facility visited by an average of 500 patients each day, but its complement of full-time medical doctors fluctuated between eight and 14. The recommended norm for rural district hospitals is one doctor to ten beds (Versteeg et al. 2013). South Africa's politics of neo-patrimonialism had also taken its toll. Newspaper reports described senior management as 'inept', 'feared by staff' and 'protected by political allies' (De Waal 2013). Senior management transferred the hospital's only HIV specialist to the out patients' department after he filed grievances against them.[17] There has also been a litany of complaints about the loss of files, constant drug shortages, patients being served rotten food, and non-functioning equipment (ibid.). Whereas Rixile's patients seldom waited for more than an hour, general visitors to the hospital commonly waited in queues from well before sunrise until late afternoon before receiving medical attention.

Many seriously ill patients came to rely on home-based care provided by unpaid volunteers. Since 2002, Hope Humana, a USAID project, has offered 25-day courses to groups of local women. These instructions cover topics such as HIV transmission, testing and treatment, prevention, risk management, positive living, nutrition, psychosocial well-being and counselling. Training also includes extensive practical sessions. The carers are well equipped to identify the symptoms of tuberculosis and AIDS, provide sick persons with assistance, and refer them to hospital when necessary. They clean the incapacitated, wash their clothes, fetch water and cook for them, tidy their homes and yards, and ensure that they take their medication as instructed. Each carer visits about 12 patients each week and maintains utmost confidentiality about their status. These volunteers are more attuned to non-biomedical discourses on misfortune and sickness than doctors and nurses might be.

Contrary to what biopolitical theory might lead us to expect, health has not been a focal point of political activism. The TAC had no political presence in Bushbuckridge, and during fieldwork I heard few complaints about President Mbeki's policies on antiretroviral drugs. HIV/AIDS simply did not feature during campaigns for the national elections of 2004 (Niehaus 2006a). On occasion, doctors threatened to stop work if government did not improve salaries and security at Tintswalo hospital. In 2012, the BRA submitted a memorandum to the Mpumalanga Health Department listing complaints about deaths and the unfair award of tenders at Tintswalo hospital (Hlatshwayo 2012). But, over time, crime has been a far more prominent focus of political mobilisation than healthcare provision (Niehaus 2012a).

Biomedical discourses on HIV/AIDS have not displaced existing beliefs in the polluting powers of death, the operation of witchcraft, and the vitality of spiritual agencies. Nor has it diminished the force of religious and political discourses on HIV/AIDS.

Organisation of the book

My arguments about the HIV/AIDS pandemic in Bushbuckridge are formulated throughout the following six chapters, entitled 'Death', 'Blame', 'Words', 'Knowledge', 'Dreams' and 'Care'. The chapters are not organised to address the concerns of biomedical and public health practitioners, but rather to capture those of ordinary people living with AIDS, their kin and associates. The chapters are roughly arranged chronologically and pertain to different periods in the historical unfolding of the pandemic and in the provision of therapy.

In Chapters 2 to 4, I address the initial phases of the pandemic, before the availability of HAART, when interventions assumed the forms of AIDS awareness that emphasised prevention. In Chapter 2, I argue that the portrayal of AIDS as an incurable sickness in public health propaganda, combined with local understandings of death as a contaminating force, produced the perception of HIV-infected persons as 'living corpses' who were dangerous to others. I suggest that, in Impalahoek, this framing, rather than the sexual mode of transmission of HIV, formed the key basis of stigma and shame. Chapter 3 examines how three sets of discourses about HIV/AIDS – public health propaganda, conspiracy theories and witchcraft accusations – configured and reconfigured blame. Public health discourses amounted to a form of victim-blaming that singled out sick persons themselves, not only for responsibility for contracting HIV, but also for culpability of having infected past and present lovers with a terminal syndrome. Hence, diagnoses of being HIV-positive have led to bitter recriminations and conflict. By contrast, village-based conspiracy theories about the origin and transmission of HIV expressed popular anxieties about the capriciousness of broader political and economic processes. In the case of witchcraft accusations, sick persons and their kin attributed the very same afflictions that biomedical doctors saw as symptomatic of HIV/AIDS to the witchcraft of kin and neighbours. In this manner, witchcraft accusations were bids to reinforce social relations of kinship and marriage that the biomedical diagnosis of being HIV-positive threatened to disrupt.

In Chapter 4, I discuss people's fear of being pronounced HIV-positive as a reason for their reluctance to undergo tests for HIV antibodies. I suggest that these beliefs express deep-rooted assumptions about the dangerous capacity of speech acts, such as cursing, to materialise disease. These assumptions are also evident in the avoidance of direct speech about sex, death and AIDS in everyday social intercourse.

In the next two chapters I focus on the period since 2005, marked by the public 'roll-out' of HAART. Although the availability of effective medication has gradually eroded the stigma of AIDS, in many domains it has not brought about the hegemony of biomedical meanings. In Chapter 5, I present the life story of Reggie Ngobeni, a man who was diagnosed HIV-positive and successfully used HAART. Reggie's experiences show the problematic status of the concept of 'knowledge' in contexts of radical therapeutic pluralism. Rather than a firm commitment to biomedical paradigms, Reggie understood his own condition through constantly shifting perspectives, and through the successive invocation of spirit possession, bewitchment and sexual pollution. In his quest for a cure, Reggie consulted a wide array of diviners, Christian healers and biomedical practitioners, but he remained uncertain about the accuracy of their diagnoses and the efficacy of their treatments. In Chapter 6, I focus more closely on local understandings of antiretroviral medication. I show that people using HAART were particularly attentive to their experience of vivid and frightening dreams and understood the meanings of these through established frameworks of dream interpretation. Whereas physicians saw dreams as a biochemical side effect of the compound efavirenz, patients themselves saw these dreams as intrinsic to the efficacy of HAART.

In Chapter 7, I examine the aftermath of AIDS and discuss the situation of orphans whose parents have died of AIDS-related diseases. I argue that Northern Sotho and Shangaan models for kinship, marked by a diffusion of parenthood, have facilitated the care and guardianship of AIDS orphans. Due to pervasive marital breakdown, and to the prerequisites for the awarding of child foster grants, the burden of care has largely fallen on women relatives, such as the orphan's sisters, mother's sisters and maternal grandmother.

In conclusion, I assess the conceptual, theoretical and political implications of these arguments, and ask how the insights they provide can aid better treatment and care. I also explore obstacles to and possibilities for understanding social and cultural difference in contemporary South Africa.

2
Death

During my visit to Impalahoek in July 2003, one of my research assistants, Ace Ubisi, was extremely upset. Ace said that his friend Platos Bila had recently died from AIDS-related diseases, and he was furious about the way in which Platos had been treated at Tintswalo hospital and by his own kin. In earlier years Platos had worked as a migrant labourer at a construction company in Johannesburg. During 1999, he became severely ill, and returned home to his wife. However, Platos's parents did not believe that he had AIDS but claimed that his wife had bewitched him. Under pressure, she returned to her natal family, and Platos was compelled to move into his parents' home. Ace believed the accusation of witchcraft was insincere and had been made on spurious grounds.

Platos used to attend hospital, but the nurses became sick and tired of treating him and sent him home. Platos's parents then brought him to live in a small room, outside their home. Some neighbours said that Platos had malaria: others said that he had AIDS. Maybe Platos had both malaria and AIDS. He was very thin and he had black spots on his legs. After four months he could no longer walk.

Platos lay on a mattress – not on a bed. He had diarrhoea and his family members no longer wanted to clean his shit. They would only enter the room once a day, hold their noses, and place one plate of food and one cup of water on the floor. I could hear Platos scream, pleading for water. His sister sometimes came from her own home to clean him and to bring him food. She said that even if her brother should die, he should die peacefully – not like an animal. This is because Platos had paid for her education. Sometimes I became angry and took him water. Then his brothers opened the door so that I could talk to him. Because it stank like hell, I would stand outside. It even stank outside where I stood.

None of Platos's friends came to his funeral. His parents did not want us to help with the arrangements. It seemed to us that his family wanted him to die early so that they could get his pension money.

Experiences such as those of Platos Bila are dramatic reminders of so many instances in which government, the biomedical fraternity and kinship networks failed to provide humane care for persons suffering from AIDS-related diseases. These experiences also demonstrate the pervasive stigma attached to this syndrome. In the words of Goffman, HIV/AIDS had extensive 'discrediting effects', which reduced 'whole and usual' persons such Platos Bila to being 'tainted and discounted' (Goffman 1971: 3).

Few social analysts have documented and accounted for the stigma of HIV/AIDS in Southern Africa. Much attention has been focused on the silence and denial that characterised the responses of President Mbeki's government to AIDS. But less often recognised is that these responses resonated with those prevailing in village and township settings throughout the country. Apart from the urban-based Treatment Action Campaign, few South Africans opposed the government's AIDS policies. This was evident during the national elections of 2004, when the ruling ANC increased its national majority and secured 69.7 per cent of all votes cast. Village and township residents have remained silent about AIDS, but have also, in certain cases, shunned, ostracised and abandoned people suffering from the syndrome (Skhosana 2001; Stein 2003). During a tragic episode that occurred in KwaZulu-Natal during 1998, men stoned to death a young woman, Gugu Dlamini, who announced publicly that she was HIV-positive. Her killers reportedly felt that she had 'shamed their community' (McNeil 1998).

Some social scientists assert that the negative cultural baggage of AIDS arises from processes of domination and exclusion. Farmer (1992) and Parker and Aggleton (2003) argue that, in the US and Europe, dominant social classes associate AIDS with marginal outsiders such as intravenous drug users, gay men, sex workers, and immigrants from Haiti and Africa. This association is not only statistical; it also reflects social prejudice against certain groups. However, the South African situation is very different. There appears to be limited 'othering' in discourses about AIDS among black citizens. In the country, HIV is mainly spread by heterosexual intercourse, and wealthier and poorer people have roughly similar risks of infection (Deacon 2002; Shisana et al. 2002).

Another approach has been to locate the stigma of AIDS in the specific local interpretations of its mode of transmission and symptoms. Previous intellectual excursions on these lines have highlighted the association of HIV infections with sexual promiscuity. For example, Posel describes President Mbeki's denial of AIDS as partly a reaction to racist renditions of Africans as 'promiscuous carriers of germs', who display 'uncontrollable devotion to the sin of lust' (2005: 143). This perception is more likely to account for AIDS denial among South Africa's ruling elite, who attach greater weight to African nationalist concerns than do commoners.[1] Ethnographic texts show South Africans to be open about heterosexuality – condoning teenage sexual exploration, accepting illegitimate children, and not allowing adultery to cause too much disruption (Delius and Glaser 2005). Ashforth writes that, in Soweto, sexual licentiousness inspires little shame:

> After all there is hardly a family in the country that does not have
> children giving birth to children, sons being sought to support
> their offspring, or fathers finding lost progeny they secretly
> sired many years back. Sexual misdemeanours are shameful,
> sometimes, but commonplace, nonetheless. (Ashforth 2002: 127)

South African men often claim that they are naturally inclined and traditionally entitled to be polygamous (Spiegel 1989) and see their capacity to have multiple sexual liaisons as a sign of masculine success (Hunter 2005).[2] Promiscuous women generally provoke greater criticism. But village and township residents acknowledge that in the context of grinding poverty women engage in 'transactional' sex in a desperate attempt to support themselves and their dependants (Wojcicki 2002). Religious conservativism seems to have had an uneven impact throughout the country. While Pentecostal churches condemn pre- and extramarital sexual intercourse, sexual morality is of marginal concern in South Africa's more numerous Zionist and Apostolic churches (Garner 2000).

For me, the interpretation of the symptoms of AIDS as indices of death appears to be a more pronounced source of its stigma. This suggestion is not entirely novel. Ashforth (2005) and Viljoen (2005) observe that residents of Hammanskraal and Soweto, respectively, describe AIDS as a 'waiting room for death' and refer to HIV-positive persons as 'dead before dying'. But neither author develops these ideas in sufficient depth.

These observations, and also Hertz's (1960 [1907]) classical analysis of death, constitute the starting point for my discussion of AIDS stigma in this chapter. Hertz argued that in many social contexts death is conceptualised not as a single event but rather as a process in which the deceased is gradually transferred from the land of the living into the realm of the dead. In this process, he argues,

'biological death', which ends the human organism, does not necessarily coincide with 'social death', which extinguishes the person's
social identity. Biological death usually precedes social death, and
in the ambiguous state between these points the deceased is in a
kind of limbo and is potentially dangerous to others. The disjuncture between biological and social death is particularly evident in
African contexts where the dead person remains an omnipresent
part of the lives of his or her kin, as an ancestor (ibid.). There are
also circumstances in which social death could precede biological
death, for example when someone is confined to an institution, such
as a hospice, for the rest of their life (Helman 1994). Bloch (1988)
develops these insights. He suggests that, in Western legal contexts,
an emphasis on the precise moment of death is an expression of
the bounded individuality of the person. Where personhood is more
diffuse and relationally constituted, death is more likely to be viewed
as a process. From this perspective, one can see that the symbolic
location of people with AIDS in an anomalous domain betwixt and
between life and death is a potent source of its stigma.

   In the sections below, I first examine how residents of Impalahoek interpreted the sexual mode of transmitting HIV and explain
why their perceptions of sexual immorality does not fully explain the
stigma of AIDS. I then argue that the perception of HIV-infected
persons as 'living corpses' (setopo sa gopela) is a far more pervasive
reason for its discrediting effects. Such labelling is not purely a
product of biomedicine; rather, it is an outcome of the way in which
public health discourses about AIDS as a terminal sickness have
articulated with popular understandings of death as a polluting force.
I endeavour to show how Christian associations of AIDS with biblical
leprosy and village-based representations of persons with AIDS as
victims of zombie-making witchcraft have coloured biomedical
meanings in a manner not predictable through biopolitical theory.

The sexual hypothesis

Residents of Impalahoek recognised sexual promiscuity as a source
of the transmission of HIV. The Tsonga euphemisms for AIDS –
sephamula ('open up') and phamukati ('lie down') – explicitly refer
to women's positions during sexual intercourse. During interviews,
I frequently heard elderly informants attribute the high incidence
of AIDS to the unscrupulous sexual conduct of the younger generation. Sitting on a reed mat, underneath the shade of a tree in her

yard, a woman pensioner told me during an interview: 'In the past we married, but today the youth have lost their morals. They ignore taboos and screw about. This is why they are dying like ants.' Such comments were common. But the recognition that husbands might infect their faithful wives, and that mothers might transmit HIV to their babies through breastfeeding, weakened the link between sexual promiscuity and AIDS, as did miasmic theories of contagion.

Sex was widely seen as a source of power that embodied opposing moral potentials. On the one hand, residents of Impalahoek perceived sex as a means of procreation and pleasure, necessary for the maintenance of good health (Collins and Stadler 2000). They suggested that heterosexual intercourse ensured a balanced mixture of blood: in the sex act, a man first injected semen (known as white blood) and then absorbed the woman's vaginal fluids (another form of blood). Getting married and bearing children were ideal attributes of adult personhood. Many men took pride in having extramarital lovers. In fact, many village adults deemed celibacy and singleness to be more dishonourable than promiscuity. They said that prolonged celibacy caused poorly regulated bodily fluids, short temper, recklessness and depression, and they were always extremely suspicious of adult male bachelors (*kgope* or *lefetwa*) who lived alone. The very same elders who complained about the loose sexual mores of youth told me that, in the past, kin could become so incensed at a man who had died without leaving progeny that they might express their discontent by shoving a burning log into the anus of his corpse.

On the other hand, villagers acknowledged that sex could also be a source of danger and immorality (Heald 1995). There was an elaborate vocabulary of sexually transmitted diseases. Sex between spouses or regular lovers, who were immune to each other, was deemed safe because their bodies regularly exchanged sweat, blood, odours and aura (*seriti*). But, in the case of incest, where patrilineal kin were of the same blood, there could be no mingling, resulting in the birth of crippled or mentally retarded babies. However, inauspicious sex could bring about an excessive mixture of substances. If a woman had made love to several men, her lovers would absorb substances from each other's bodies via her body. Should any man who had been polluted in this manner contact children, those children could contract an affliction called *makgoma* (*kgoma*, 'to touch') and experience convulsions and shortness of breath.

The most commonly recognised sexually transmitted diseases were gonorrhoea (*toropo*) and syphilis (*leshofela*). There were also other afflictions that arose when men had sexual intercourse with women who were pregnant, with widows, or with women who had recently aborted. In local belief, such women were in a dangerous state of multiplicity, conceptualised as heat (*fiša*). The bodies of pregnant women constituted a duality between mother and foetus; and those of widows and women who had recently aborted were contaminated by the aura (*seriti*) of the deceased husband or aborted foetus. Any man who had intercourse with such women would contract an affliction called 'shudder' (*lešiši*). Their heat might cause his entire body to swell up and his groin to ache so badly that he might be unable to walk. In the case of abortion, his blood would be poisoned; he would be unable to urinate, and he would sweat profusely and cough severely.

The transgression of sexual taboos undoubtedly coloured people's understandings of HIV/AIDS, but it seems implausible that the association of AIDS with these dangerous kinds of sexual intercourse alone might explain its stigma. There was a significant disjuncture between immoral and dangerous sexual activities. Many residents of Impalahoek perceived masturbation and homosexuality as highly immoral (Niehaus 2002c), but they did not view these as routes for transmitting HIV. The belief of a male research participant who had worked in the Witwatersrand mines for many years clearly contradicted biomedical knowledge. He said that some of his peers engaged in male-to-male sex while they resided in the mining compounds, precisely because they perceived it to be hygienic:

> I have personally asked the elderly men why they prefer [to have sex with] boys. They tell me that women bite. They say that a woman can make you ill and give you STDs [sexually transmitted diseases]. You can even die if she had committed an abortion. With women, there is also AIDS. They say it is safe with a young boy. He won't transfer any diseases to you.

In the moral economy of sexuality, young women who eloped with lovers attracted more condemnatory remarks than young men who engaged in multiple sexual liaisons. Because no bridewealth had been paid, such liaisons subverted the authority of the woman's parents. Yet young women were more likely than young men to take tests for HIV antibodies, undergo counselling, and join support groups for persons living with AIDS at the Rixile clinic.

Moreover, the sexual route of transmission does not explain silence and discreet talk about AIDS in the public domain. Talk about sex was proscribed. Elders, particularly parents, were prohibited from speaking directly to younger people about sex, and vice versa. Instead, it was the mother's brother (*malome*) and younger sister (*mangwane*) who were expected to educate their nephews and nieces about sexual matters. Grandparents also joked with grandchildren about sex, in a non-reciprocal manner. In these forms of talk, sex was referred to indirectly, by euphemisms such as to 'share a blanket' (*ke lepai re ya apolelana*), 'penetrate' (*tobetsa*), 'taste' (*kwa*), 'perform' (*maka*) or 'sleep' (*robala*). The most open and direct talk about sex occurred between spouses, lovers, coevals and friends, and between villagers and relative outsiders such as anthropologists. Cousins shared a reciprocal joking relationship in which they frequently shared lewd sexual jokes.

With respect to silence, AIDS differed significantly from other STDs. Male research participants freely told me about how they had personally suffered from gonorrhoea, syphilis and *lešiši*. They said that any husband who had contracted an STD was expected to tell his wife, so that they, together, could consult diviners to seek a cure. In the case of *lešiši*, which was potentially fatal, a man also had to inform his uncles and aunts. A middle-aged man who had once contracted this affliction during his youth explained to me: 'If you do not speak out you might breathe your last breath.' Women perceived STDs as more shameful. But, according to women research participants, women, too, regularly spoke about these conditions at women's clubs and associations.

It seems to me that the key difference that accounted for the silence surrounding AIDS was its terminal nature, at least in the years before antiretroviral treatment was available. Residents of Impalahoek were confident that diviners and biomedical practitioners could easily cure other sexually transmitted diseases and afflictions. The Sotho-speaking Malopo spirits reportedly conferred those whom they possessed with special powers to diagnose and treat gonorrhoea, syphilis and *lešiši*. By boiling tree roots in water, and using this concoction to purify the blood of their clients, diviners could cure these diseases in a matter of two or three days. To treat *lešiši*, they placed a clay pot containing herbs and glowing embers on the client's head and administered enemas to make him discharge thick blood.

AIDS as death

The association of AIDS with dying and with death is a more likely source of its stigma, and illuminates many aspects of people's responses to AIDS. In interviews, research participants generally spoke of AIDS as a most dreadful untreatable and fatal illness, resulting in a most horrible death. This is expressed in the following statements about the fears that men had of being diagnosed HIV-positive.

> If you test HIV-positive you will lose your memory, thinking all the time about death and dying. People will not gossip about you because you screw, but because you are dead. They will take you as dead. They will take you as a living corpse.

> We Blacks [black people], we are brought up to believe that death is a terrible tragedy. If they tell me that I am HIV-positive, I'll think of dying. I'll automatically think that I'm dead. I will see death. Because people fear death so much they would not want to talk to me or even come close to me.

Such exaggerations were a product of the way in which public health activists and Christian ministers alike labelled AIDS as a terminal illness, and of how biomedical and religious discourses articulated with popular, village-based, understandings of death.

During the 1990s, public health propaganda actively, although not always intentionally, associated AIDS with death. The scale and urgency of AIDS awareness campaigns throughout Bushbuckridge vastly exceeded that of previous initiatives on malaria, tuberculosis and family planning. Through excessive propaganda to stem the spread of HIV, the campaigns created the impression that AIDS was somehow deadlier than other diseases. Moreover, by focusing on prevention rather than cure, they created the impression that because AIDS is incurable, it is also untreatable, and that little can be done to assist anyone who is HIV-positive. These messages came too late, at a time when many villagers had already been infected or considered themselves to have been infected with the virus.

AIDS awareness activists employed by the Health Systems Development Unit, Reproductive Health Groups Project, Bushbuckridge Health and Social Service Consortium (BHSSC) and LoveLife Y-Centre adopted this approach. LoveLife educators were known for the scary tactics they deployed. A young man who was particularly interested in the computer training offered by the Y-Centre told me that he also frequently attended other organised events. At one workshop, he recalled, the attendants were told that AIDS is incurable, and they were shown a videocassette of Ethiopians dying of

AIDS-related diseases. He said that the only message they received about treatment was that those who ate fruit and vegetables might prolong their lives.

Aaron Dlamini, who once worked as a paid AIDS awareness activist for LoveLife (called a 'groundbreaker' in institutional jargon), made similar telling criticisms of the organisation's strategy:

> I worked at LoveLife because I wanted a job and I only did what I was told. I had to tell people 'AIDS kills! Use condoms!' ... We only talked about prevention. We said AIDS was incurable. That is why we must prevent it. We never told people what to do [if they were infected]. People who go around with the awareness put a bad stigma on AIDS. They will say that AIDS kills. I think every disease kills: also, high blood, diabetes and tuberculosis.[3] Why don't they do blood pressure awareness? People have guns and guns kill. They don't have gun awareness. Guns are meant to kill!

But even youngsters who were uninterested in LoveLife could not escape these messages. As elsewhere in South Africa (Gallant and Maticka-Tyndale 2004), AIDS awareness soon became an integral component of 'life orientation' classes in all Bushbuckridge schools. Each quarter, teachers of Impalahoek primary school divided the learners into three groups for AIDS awareness classes: children between eight and 12, boys older than 12, and girls older than 12. Teachers did not mention sex to the younger children, but warned them not to play with scissors, razors and pins; not to touch bleeding friends; and not to inflate any balloons (condoms) they found lying about in the village streets. (These lessons propagated miasmic theories of contagion.) Teachers taught the older learners the ABC – to Abstain, Be faithful and Condomise – and demonstrated safe sex with stage props such as artificial penises and various kinds of condoms. AIDS activists targeted high schools for even more excessive propaganda, and in some instances they addressed high school learners as often as twice a week. The instructions were mainly about prevention but also mentioned the benefits of voluntary counselling and testing, of medication, and of a healthy diet. Younger people were over-saturated with these messages.

This period also saw a proliferation of religious discourses that imposed a moralist reading of HIV/AIDS. Ministers of the 27 churches of Impalahoek portrayed the pandemic as divine retribution for sin: not only for individuals having unprotected sex, but also for a world that had gone morally astray. The ministers pointed to escalating violent crimes throughout the country, to corrupt nationalist politicians who enriched themselves at the expense of the electorate, to youth who disrespected elders, and to the legalisation of gay marriage and abortion. I occasionally heard ministers and senior church members refer to HIV/AIDS as a new kind of leprosy. They either posited a metaphorical relationship between these conditions, or else identified skin lesions (an opportunistic infection associated with AIDS) as leprosy. Although isolated cases of leprosy did occur in Bushbuckridge until the 1970s, few villagers were acquainted with the clinical details of the condition. They nonetheless described leprosy as a most contagious illness and portrayed lepers as maximally ravaged, horribly deformed people, whose flesh literally rotted away while they were still alive. This trope clearly derives from biblical mythology, pertaining to Leviticus, in which the leper was 'tainted with death' and 'carried in his person a defiling taint which excluded him absolutely from any contact with holy things, even contact with clean people, even contact with the community' (Lewis 1987: 596).[4]

Christians seemed to believe that AIDS was somehow deadlier that ordinary leprosy. While they portrayed AIDS as terminal, they readily cited biblical passages showing how God and Jesus had cured lepers. Another difference was that symptoms of AIDS were, initially, invisible. But invisibility provided little comfort. In the villages of Bushbuckridge, where the secret, sinister powers of witchcraft were a 'standardised nightmare' (Wilson 1951), the concealed generally inspired greater anxiety and fear than the transparent.

These biomedical and religious discourses on HIV/AIDS intersected with vernacular perceptions and modes of treating terminally ill persons, death and bereavement. Until the late 1960s, close adult relatives of the deceased buried his or her corpse inside the yard on the very same evening as death. But since then, these processes have become far more ritualised and dramatic. During the early 1970s, the government established mortuaries and built public graveyards. Mortuaries enabled families to stretch the liminal period between death and burial (Van der Geest 2006) and to undertake elaborate preparations for hosting grand funerals on Saturdays. Funerals now regularly drew attendances of more than 500 people and became the single most important space for kin and neighbours to express social concern and enact moral solidarity (Durham and Klaits 2002; Lee 2011).

Much like biblical lepers who were tainted with death, villagers conceptually located terminally ill people in an anomalous domain, betwixt and between life and death. This is apparent in the term 'noisy ancestors' (*bakwale badimo*) that was sometimes applied to them. Villagers treated terminally ill persons as socially dead, while physically still alive, and secluded them from neighbours. This practice was observed with such regularity that one middle-aged male research participant told me that he had never seen a dying person. 'They always hide them away,' he remarked. Only a few select people could nurse the terminally ill. Traditionally, nursing was gendered. A father nursed his son, a mother her daughter, a married person his or her spouse, a brother or younger paternal uncle (*rangwane*) a widower, and a sister or younger maternal aunt (*mangwane*) a widow. But due to the vagaries of the migrant labour system and pervasive marital breakdown, it was usually mothers who washed, fed and cared for the sick. The proverb 'The child's mother holds the knife by its sharp end' (*Mmago ngwana o swara tipa ba bogale*) alludes to the hardships any mother is prepared to undergo to protect her children.

A constantly burning fire in the yard indicated sickness within a homestead. Nobody could enter the sick person's room without the primary caregiver's permission – especially not anyone who might be polluted by birth, sex and death. People who had come from diviners or from church were also prohibited from entering the room because the medicinal prescriptions they used might counteract the sick person's medicines. Relatives and neighbours were, nonetheless, encouraged to visit the household, fetch water for them, and donate food for the sick person, without entering the room.

One of the most striking aspects of people's attitudes was their intense unease, fear or even abhorrence of a terminally ill person. Nearly all research participants said that they felt more disturbed by a 'living corpse' (*setopo sa gopela*) than by a deceased person. Despite being in a situation of extreme vulnerability and dependence, dying people were somehow seen to be dangerous. Being anomalous to the categories of 'life' and 'death', they contradicted usual schemes of classification (Douglas 1970). One research participant also described terminally ill persons as pitiful and burdensome:

> I can tolerate a corpse, but not a person who is dying. When I look at such a person his agony will be transferred to me and I will feel his pain. I will be traumatised. I will also think about those who have to care for me when I'm in such a situation.

Elderly research participants reminded me that euthanasia was common in the past.[5] This was especially the case with masters of circumcision lodges, who reportedly ate food such as tortoise hearts to ensure strength and longevity. Even though the initiation master's brain might be dead and his body rotting, his heart would continue beating. To relieve him (and others) of pain, relatives would wrap his body in blankets, place it at the entrance of the cattle kraal, and then drive the herd of cattle over him. Other means of euthanasia included placing *tshipi* herbs underneath the pillows of dying people, making them inhale *fofotsa* (also used to terminate the life of sick animals), or treating them with a mixture of fig and python-tail fat. In 2015, members of the Mashile family sprinkled herbs, obtained from a diviner, in the room of their grandmother, to ensure that she could pass on peacefully to the world of the ancestors. She was reportedly more than 100 years old. The grandmother had been bed-ridden after she broke her foot and spinal cord during a fall and could no longer eat or defecate without the assistance of her daughter-in-law. Her descendants decided to bring an end to her suffering after she repeatedly passed out, only to revive.

Whereas terminally ill people were secluded and unseen, adults were occasionally called upon to identify the corpses of relatives at mortuaries, and they regularly viewed corpses at night vigils. Corpses did not inspire nearly as much unease as dying persons but did have the capacity to pollute. Upon death, I was told, the breath (*moya*) and aura (*seriti*; literally 'shadow') of a deceased person separated from his or her corporeal body (*mmele*). The aura assumed a dark, sorrowful form called *thefifi*, which could contaminate any object, item or person that it touched. Villagers believed that a deceased person's clothes and utensils literally 'had his body' (*O na le mmele ya ka*).[6]

In cases of death, residents of Impalahoek generally followed the following procedures; there were only minor variations and exceptions. Mourners usually took great care to avoid contaminative exposure. Kin immediately took the corpse to the mortuary, where they thoroughly washed and cleansed it. The bereaved family then observed a week-long period of mourning. They erected a large tent in the yard, and the entire household slept outside their home to display their sorrow. Members of the bereaved family observed various prohibitions. They abstained from sexual intercourse, stopped working in the fields and refrained from touching children. If a member of the family was not at home at the time of death, he should enter through the main gate facing backwards and drink water from a wooden spoon. Visitors were not allowed to take any items from the homes of bereaved families. Each evening before sunset, neighbours and friends visited and consoled the bereaved family.

Late on the Friday afternoon people fetched the corpse from the mortuary and placed it inside the homestead of the bereaved family. Here, widows – who had previously been exposed to the dangers of death – prepared the corpse for a final time. To minimise its heat, they sprinkled ash on all windows. Being white, and having survived the flames of fire, ash was a prominent cooling substance, frequently used in healing rites (Hammond-Tooke 1981: 145). Mourners then held an all-night vigil, which was marked by the singing of hymns, the saying of prayers, and by short speeches to comfort the bereaved family.

On the Saturday morning, a funeral service was conducted at the home of the bereaved family. There were further recollections of the deceased, and more hymns and prayers, from speakers representing various categories of kin, affines, neighbours, friends, professional and political associations, and different churches.

Finally, a hearse transported the coffin to the graveyard. Young men usually placed items – such as blankets, walking sticks, cups and plates that had been polluted by the aura of the deceased – inside the grave. Throughout the proceedings, the widow covered her head with a blanket. A burial society then served all attendants with food at the home of the deceased. At the gate, men sprinkled everyone who entered the yard with water – on both their front and back – to cool them. After the meal, women thoroughly cleansed all the deceased's utensils. To remove all misfortune from the home, Zionist ministers sprinkled all members of the bereaved family with holy water, and cleansed the yard and all rooms with a mixture of water, milk, ash and salt. This was done to 'tie the spirit or breath' (*hlema moya*) of the deceased. However, widows were still perceived as polluting and had to observe a year-long mourning period. Children were cleansed with paraffin to immunise them against the widow's heat. Without this they might develop the affliction, *mafulara*, marked by profuse coughing.

The intersection of public health and religious discourse on HIV/AIDS with local modes of conceptualising and relating to terminal illness and death goes some way towards explaining why residents of Impalahoek viewed HIV-positive persons as 'dead before dying' and as emitting polluting heat.

Stigma of the living corpse

In local perceptions HIV/AIDS, unlike other terminal illnesses, was marked by a peculiar compression of time. The very gradual progression from infection to illness to death that so frequently characterised this condition did not seem to be culturally elaborated. Rather, the symbolic load of labelling seemed so overpowering that even persons newly infected with HIV were immediately seen as tainted with death. There was also a moral aspect to AIDS. Victims were blameworthy for having brought the disease onto themselves and were culpable of having infected their sexual partners with an inevitably fatal illness.

Research participants described AIDS, much like biblical leprosy, as marked by an anomalous mixture of living and dead flesh, and they said that the bodies of people with AIDS literally decomposed while they were still alive. This perception was common and was shared by those with little acquaintance with AIDS, as well as by persons who were infected. In conversation with me, an unemployed man expressed the following opinion:

> In the final stages AIDS is so dangerous. It is as if your flesh dies, whilst your body is still alive. Your flesh will just fall off and the bones remain. It is also as if there is no blood in your body.

My former field assistant, Jimmy Mohale, articulated similar views at the time when he was critically ill, only two weeks before his death. Jimmy suffered from both pneumonia and tuberculosis. Although Jimmy was convinced that paternal relatives had bewitched him, several of his friends told me that his body displayed many familiar symptoms of AIDS-related diseases. Lying on his bed, Jimmy complained to me that he felt cold, powerless and paralysed; and that he could neither walk nor see properly. While he breathed shallowly, he spoke with a shivering voice:

> The Jimmy that you did research with had only half a life. This life came from my maternal family. I only have ancestors on my maternal side. I am dead on my paternal side … People around here know me as being dead. That is why I don't have to be seen. You are speaking to a dead person.

Mutual acquaintances told me that, during the last few weeks of Jimmy's life, there were rumours throughout Impalahoek that he had already died. 'One can say that he died before the actual death.'

In local knowledge, the symptoms of AIDS were indices of death. Foremost among these were the skin lesions or 'black spotted marks' that appeared in the latter stages of sickness. Research participants also frequently mentioned persistent diarrhoea, constant vomiting and coughing – which indicated the loss of flesh, aura and breath – as

well as swollen glands, mouth sores and soft, fluffy hair. Persons with
AIDS themselves were greatly concerned with weight loss. A woman
research participant recalled that when her sickness was most severe
she wore two dresses, one on top of the other, to make her appear 'a
little bit thicker'. Boniness is the most pronounced feature of a corpse.
The emphasis on hair loss, too, is significant. A haircut was an essential act in rites of transition. During funerals, elderly women shaved
the deceased person's hair, and placed it inside the coffin alongside
the body. Research participants also spoke of the progressive loss of
bodily functions and of reason. For example, a man who suspected
that he might be infected with HIV explained to me that his extrem-
ities became numb, and that he no longer experienced sensations in
his fingers and toes. He also covered his body with blankets, even
though others told him it was exceptionally hot outside.

Patients and their therapy management groups sometimes utilised
the services of diviners and of Christian healers, especially when they
suspected that witchcraft was operative as a cause of sickness. Like
AIDS, witchcraft did not seem amenable to treatment by clinical
medicine (see Chapter 3). These specialists sometimes interpreted
the symptoms of the sick person as evidence that witches were trying
to capture them. They alleged that the witches first took hold of the
victim's aura, and then, progressively, of different body parts, until
they possessed the entire body. But witches deceived the victim's kin
by leaving a lifeless image of him or her behind. The kin, believing that
the victim was dead, would bury what they assumed to be his or her
body, but which was instead the stem of a fern tree that had merely
been given the victim's image. Meanwhile, at home, in a second
world, witches transformed their victims into nocturnal servants or
zombies (*ditlotlwane*), the quintessential 'living dead' of the South
African lowveld. They would cut the tongues of their victims and
reduce them to a metre tall, thereby rendering them mute, sexless,
and devoid of human desires. Witches allegedly hid any zombies they
owned during the daytime but employed them as servants at night,
compelling them to perform mindless tasks at home.

This alternative construction created some hope of treatment. For
example, when Sipho Mbolwane became bed-ridden from sickness,
a diviner told his kin that witches had captured parts of his body. The
diviner rubbed an ointment into Sipho's skin to make him invisible
to the witches at night, and brought him to an empty riverbed. (The
location presumably signified the border between life and death.)
Here, the diviner tried to retrieve Sipho's aura from the witches, by
beating drums (*dingomane*) for his ancestors, blowing a rhebok horn

and calling out his name. Sipho's kin were hopeful that he would survive, but he passed away only one week later.

Carers and others generally overestimated the contagiousness of AIDS. Hardly anyone trusted the biomedical pronouncement that people could transmit HIV only through sexual intercourse. In local belief, one could also contract the virus by sharing the sick person's toilet or cutlery, by nursing him or her without wearing latex gloves, or by contacting his or her germs, blood or breath. An archetypical story was of an elderly woman who had nursed her sick daughter, and then died of similar symptoms seven years later. This alludes to fears of the pollution of death, and to the manner in which AIDS violates the integrity of the body's boundaries.

These perceptions underlay excessive avoidance behaviour. Teachers told me that they observed how pupils refused to play with the children of AIDS victims at school. Doris Mathebula, a young woman, greeted her friends by hugging them. But one of them turned and walked away. She had apparently heard that Doris had been diagnosed as HIV-positive. At home, relatives and fellow household members tended to avoid using any of the same utensils as persons with AIDS. A cup, they said, might be affected through germs from the sick person's mouth sores. In the beginning of the pandemic, some funeral parlours wrapped the corpses of AIDS victims in plastic bags and warned family members not to open them, and not to touch the corpses before burial. Men were also known to have burned the clothes they inherited from the victims of AIDS-related diseases.

Kin took extreme care to seclude people with AIDS. This was done as much to protect the sick person from others as other people from her or him. A teacher frequently tried to visit the terminally ill sister of a colleague but was always told that she had gone to live with relatives elsewhere. However, he discovered that they had lied to him. 'All the time,' he said, 'she was right there, in the house.' Persons with AIDS also lived in self-imposed isolation. While my research assistants and I visited Michael Ngoni, who operated a small *spaza* store (a small informal grocery), we heard Christian songs faintly being sung in the house next door. Michael told us that his neighbour had AIDS and hardly ever ventured outdoors. She would only open the door when she was sure that it was her mother who had knocked. Her husband and daughter had both deserted her to live elsewhere, claiming that she was insane.

Only late during sickness did patients and their therapy management groups consult biomedical practitioners.[7] This is understandable because, until the availability of antiretroviral treatment in 2005, medical facilities for persons with AIDS were woefully inadequate. Therapy comprised testing for HIV antibodies, counselling, and treatment of AIDS-related diseases. The best treatment option they could hope for was palliative care of a relatively inferior quality, and fatalism thrived in this context. Persons with AIDS were seldom hospitalised for more than a few weeks, and mainly used clinical services on an outpatient basis. Due to the extreme stigma of AIDS, these therapeutic consultations were often secretive. Lakios Rampiri, who worked as a telephone exchange operator at the nearest hospital, recalled that his neighbours woke him very late one evening and asked him to take their sister to the outpatients' department by car. During the short journey to the hospital, they covered the sick woman's head with a blanket, as if she were a widow at a funeral. The act also seemed to express a fear that she might have contaminated others.

The care and nursing of people with AIDS aimed to re-humanise sick persons whose bodies were slowly decaying. It was portrayed as an act of love, motivated by a deep sense of moral obligation towards kin, and, often, by Christian commitment (Livingston 2012: 93–118). In Impalahoek, the ideal of gender-specific care was not always possible. Mothers, sisters and daughters, but sometimes also husbands, cared for sick women; while fathers, male cousins and maternal nephews, but sometimes also mothers, sisters and wives, cared for terminally ill men.

The care of sick men, especially men who were estranged from wives and children, was problematic, and, at times, was relegated to younger male relatives. Givens Thobela told me that he took two years off school to assist his frail grandmother to nurse his maternal uncle (*malome*). Givens fed and cleansed his uncle, and when his uncle became unable to walk, he pushed him in a wheelbarrow to the nearest clinic, more than a kilometre away. Givens was extremely worried about the gossip of neighbours and asked a professional nurse to explain to them that, because she had issued him with latex gloves, his sick uncle could not infect him with HIV.

Joseph Ngobeni, a research participant who was in his mid-twenties, recounted that his elder paternal uncle (*ramogolo*), Daniel, who was a medical doctor at Tintswalo hospital, asked him and his wife to care for his cousin, Tshepo. (Tshepo's parents were both deceased.) His uncle told them that Tshepo had tuberculosis, and promised to provide them with medication, food, and a monthly stipend of R400 each. However, Joseph told me that, from the start, he suspected that Tshepo had AIDS.

Each day at 5 [a.m.] I had to give Tsepo five different tablets.
My uncle, Daniel, did not tell me what they were for, but I saw
'ART' and 'VIRUS GUARD' written on their labels. I became
so scared. I took the tablets to the doctor and the nurses at the
Rixile [the HIV clinic] and asked them what they were for. They
also did not tell me, but asked me to bring Tsepo for a blood test.
Then, they said, they could write a letter to the social workers
so that he could get a [disability] pension. I was very scared. I
thought that maybe I was also HIV-positive. I asked my uncle
[ramogolo], if I would be infected if Tshepo was HIV-positive. But
he said that I would be okay if I didn't have wounds and if our
blood did not mix.

Joseph said that a professional nurse sometimes helped him and
his wife wash Tshepo, and that members of Tshepo's church occasionally came to their home to pray for him. He described his cousin's
symptoms in detail, alluding to his status betwixt and between life
and death.

Tshepo was very thin, his mouth was bleeding and he had
diarrhoea all the time. If he slept on his left side, we had to
turn him around. We also had to feed him with our own hands.
Tshepo used to shit like hell and we could only clean him when
he was naked and wore no underwear. He was a living corpse.
We sometimes thought he was dead. When he slept, his mouth
and eyes would be open. His ankles also straightened so his legs
became like sticks. He was losing skin because he scratched himself
so much. Some weeks he would only wake up for a few minutes.
When you spoke to him you felt as if you were irritating him.

Tshepo died in 2004. Three months later, Joseph and his wife
were still haunted by recollections of Tshepo's condition.

Poverty, labour migration and household disintegration severely
undermined the quality of palliative care. Conny Nyathi, a home-
based carer trained by the BHSSC, told me of several instances
in which sick persons were abandoned by spouses and kin. In one
case, Conny said a woman and her three children refused to nurse
her husband, whom they accused of witchcraft. In another, she told
me of two brothers whose wives had abandoned them. Although
they lived with their mother, she refused to wash them, because she
did not wish to see them naked. They had both soiled their beds
and the older brother's penis had retracted into his pelvis. Conny

was shocked, not only by the severity of their discomfort but also by the failure of their kin to live up to their obligation to provide care. She recalled:

> I used water, a large basin and soap to clean [the men and their bedding] and I helped the older brother bathe. He could not go to the toilet and I let him defecate in a small bucket and poured it down the pit latrine. I did not want to go there [to the home] again, but I did. On my way, I started to cry. I told myself, 'I'm not doing it for those people, I'm doing it for God.' The one brother asked me, 'Why are you so kind to us?' I replied, 'I'm just helping you because you are unable.'

In very isolated cases, sick people died alone. Moses Selinda, who was a chronic alcoholic, lived by himself in a three-room RDP (Reconstruction and Development Programme) home and earned a living by repairing shoes. After Moses became seriously ill, he was admitted to the tuberculosis ward of Tintswalo hospital, but he was later discharged. In 2002, after neighbours complained of the stench at his home, police broke open the door, and found that Moses had been dead for nearly five days.

As the AIDS pandemic claimed more lives, surviving relatives started to hold funeral services earlier in the morning, sometimes well before sunrise. This seemed to be an attempt to pre-empt outsiders, who were not immediate kin, from attending.

Conclusions

To summarise, in Impalahoek HIV-infected persons encountered extensive stigma. They were spoken of as tainted and discredited people, whose proximity simultaneously provoked sympathy, anxiety and fear of contaminative exposure. They were secluded from fellow villagers, and were, on some occasions, ostracised, mistreated and abandoned. I suggest that these negative perceptions were not simply attributed to the association of AIDS with sexual promiscuity, but rather to the status of HIV-positive persons as 'living corpses' who were 'tainted with death'. Such labelling is evident in the perception that the bodies of persons with AIDS were literally decomposing and rotting away while they were still alive, and in their conceptual association with lepers and zombies. Like leprosy, AIDS was defined as a maximal horrible sickness (Gussow and Tracy 1977), and, like zombies, they exhibited an anomalous status in respect to the realms of the living and the dead (Niehaus 2005).

This argument has important implications. First, it points to a serious imbalance in the literature on HIV/AIDS: whereas most researchers in this area examine the ways in which people view and speak about sex and sexuality, few have explored local interpretations of AIDS-related sicknesses.[8] This is understandable, given the grim and emotionally taxing nature of the latter task. Researchers, too, have remained in their comfort zones, keeping silent about the more disturbing aspects of AIDS. Yet it is precisely in this relatively unexplored terrain that its stigma resides.

Second, and more importantly for the purpose of our argument here, the ethnographic evidence that I have presented suggests that such labelling was the result of a far more complex entanglement of biomedical, public health and religious discourses, together with vernacular understandings of terminal illness, than biopolitical theory might suggest. In this assemblage of discourses, it is virtually impossible to disentangle global discourses from local ones. In his perceptive study of Papua New Guinea, Eves (2012) reminds us that religious understandings of HIV/AIDS may well be as transnational in their remit as biomedical ones. Before the availability of anti-retroviral drugs in Impalahoek, biomedical categories did not form the basis for assertions to rights and political activism (Petryna 2002), nor did it constitute grounds and 'economies of hope' (Rose 2001: 7). Instead, the biomedical presentation of HIV/AIDS as a terminal condition, with little prospect of recovery, promoted stigma, silence and fatalism.

Third, the incapacity of biomedicine to deal effectively with AIDS-related diseases created special scope for non-biological discourses. This is especially pertinent to modes of practice pertaining to terminal illness and death in the domestic domain. The extreme unease that terminal illness inspired, and anxieties that the aura of the deceased might pollute mourners, was crucial to the stigma of AIDS, as was the dramatisation of death in highly elaborate public funerals throughout Southern Africa.

3
Blame

On 7 August 2008, Ace Ubisi and I accompanied May Mokoena, one of the very few local HIV-positive AIDS awareness activists, and Loisy Phatudi, his girlfriend, to a specially arranged workshop for the teaching staff of Shatale high school. A handsome man in his mid-thirties, May had tested HIV-positive and registered a CD4 count of only 29 in 2005. By now, ARV drugs were available, and nurses placed him on a regime of stavudine, lamivudine and stocktin. May's health improved dramatically, and by 2007 his CD4 count was 781. He had become an activist for an NGO called Obrigado ('thank you' in Portuguese) out of a sense of religious obligation, but also as a desperate means of earning a living. May was an exceptionally good speaker.

His message to the 23 teachers, at various grades of seniority, was a very positive one, emphasising the possibility of healing after so many years of despair. However, May began his talk by drawing an elaborate, hypothetical, sexual network on the chalk board. Nearly all sexual partners in the network engaged in extramarital affairs, and, in his words, 'cheated each other'. A hypothetical man named Rodney, who resided in Shatale, infected a couple called Frida and Vincient, in Middelburg. They, in turn, spread HIV to Maria and Jack in Cape Town. The virus was then transmitted to Joyce and Victor in Durban, Rebecca and Mpo in Witbank, Phandy and Joe in Hazyview, Ruth and Aaron in Bushbuckridge, and finally to Rodney's own sister, Monica, in Shatale. 'Protect yourselves,' May said. 'You might unintentionally infect your own family.' The teachers seemed to be particularly attentive to his narrative. For them, May's talk provided a welcome break from the pressure of their everyday work routine. They also valued the opportunity to hear someone speak openly about AIDS, and to see, touch and inspect the ARV drugs that May distributed.

The workshop, nonetheless, left a bitter aftertaste. Like countless other well-intentioned AIDS awareness initiatives, May's message contained a 'persecutorial' view of misfortune (Taylor 1992: 62). It reinforced the perception that HIV-positive people were unwise in their sexual choices and practices,[1] responsible for their own sickness, and also culpable for spreading the virus to others. Such victim-blaming divided target audiences on the basis of a disreputable alterity and contributed to the exclusion of persons living with AIDS from networks of social interaction.

The attribution of responsibility and blame has been a central feature of epidemics throughout history. Rosenberg (1992) argues that epidemics are 'social sampling devices' that 'strip life bare' to reveal ideas, structural inequalities and conflicts that are kept subdued in less critical times. In Europe, citizens were historically inclined to single out foreigners and Jews as disease carriers, and in India they treated 'untouchables' as scapegoats for epidemics (see Herring and Swelund 2010). Similarly, the AIDS pandemic spawned complex 'geographies of blame' (Farmer 1992). In the global North, epidemiologists labelled disreputable populations, such as Haitian immigrants, as 'risk groups', and in the global South, popular discourses blamed European sex tourists for introducing HIV. Within village communities throughout the world, men blamed 'free women' and elders the youth for spreading the disease (Weiss 1993).

In this chapter, I investigate the configuration and reconfiguration of blame for HIV/AIDS in Impalahoek, particularly during the initial stages of the HIV/AIDS pandemic. I suggest that the attribution of blame has been the product of diverse and divergent discourses that articulate interests and concerns existing outside the domains of sickness and healing. These discourses include: (1) public health propaganda about the sexual transmission of HIV/AIDS; (2) popular conspiracy theories on the origin and spread of HIV that circulated within the village setting; and (3) accusations of witchcraft that occurred largely at the level of individual households. In the sections below, I outline the contents of each of these discourses, their social bases, and their mutual entanglements.

Far from exhibiting a narrow and depoliticising objectivist focus on somatic categories (Taussig 1980; Kleinman 1995), I argue that public health discourses in Impalahoek rapidly became deeply enmeshed in local social relations, particularly those pertaining to gender. They were most eagerly embraced by women, who blamed authoritarian, sometimes violent, men for intentionally spreading the virus to their lovers. These accusations generated bitter conflict on lines of gender. In the next sections of the chapter, I suggest that both conspiracy theories and witchcraft accusations contested victim-blaming inherent in public health discourses. Although conspiracy theories[2] were multi-layered and contradictory, they allocated responsibility for the pandemic to forces – such as government and big business – located well beyond the village setting. They were narrated largely by men, who framed discussions about HIV/AIDS in terms of political paradigms. Their narrative intentions were shaped by their increasingly anxious encounters in South Africa's industrial centres as labour migrants. The gendered nature of these discourses seemed to reinforce the dictum that women are to men as the local is to the global (Freeman 2001).

In the final part of the chapter, I aim to show that whereas outsiders such as neighbours were inclined to mention AIDS when talking behind the scenes, carers and close kin were more likely to identify witchcraft as the cause of specific deaths. This concurs with studies that detect links between the HIV/AIDS pandemic and a resurgence of witchcraft accusations and witchcraft eradication movements elsewhere in sub-Saharan Africa.[3] According to classical theory, as an ideational system witchcraft provides a logical explanation for the particularities of misfortune, and answers the central questions 'Why him or her?' and 'Why now?' (Evans-Pritchard 1937). But in the case of HIV/AIDS, I argue, we can also see the invocation of witchcraft as a bid to reconfigure culpability, absolve victims of blame, and redraw the boundaries of networks of sociability.

Biomedicine, gender and the politics of blame

AIDS awareness campaigns had a deep impact in Impalahoek. Yet the interviews that Gunvor Jonnson and I conducted with the help of our research assistants in 2002 and 2005 revealed a gendered difference in receptivity to public health propaganda.

Women were generally most knowledgeable about, and committed to, biomedical discourses on HIV/AIDS. This resonates with their orientation towards the 'ways of whites' (sekgowa)[4] and the medicalisation of women's bodies through gynaecological examinations (Martin 1992). Young women invested in schooling and in church activities and committed themselves to monogamous marriage. Moreover, their leisure time activities included reading magazines, watching soap operas on television, and listening to radio – all forums for discussions of HIV/AIDS.

Despite the long history of mistrust and resistance to colonial health services and medical interventions in the field of fertility (Hunt 1999; White 2000: 81–121), women acknowledged the expertise of nurses and doctors. Some young women learned about AIDS from LoveLife groundbreakers who addressed life orientation classes at school, or from the media. Others were told of AIDS when they underwent prenatal examinations. One interviewee, Joyce Ubisi, told Gunvor Jonnson that she distrusted friends as sources of information and that she regretted that she had not heard sooner about AIDS from 'professionals'.

Women distinguished between AIDS and *mafulara* (an affliction caused by the transgression of funeral taboos). They described HIV/AIDS as a virus contained in blood, semen and vaginal fluids, which was transmitted by sexual intercourse. Young women commented that one could also contract HIV from touching blood if one had a scratch, and by using contaminated injection needles. They also believed that pregnant women could transmit AIDS to their babies through breastfeeding. Their only blatantly incorrect response was that one could contract HIV by 'kissing boys with AIDS'.

Young women generally preferred condoms to birth control injections, which they claimed made them fat and caused excessive menstruation. Patricia Mashile, who had recently completed school, said: 'I trust condoms. The solution to AIDS is that we must talk about it and put on condoms. I will tell my son about condoms when he is seven years old.' Her friend, Iris Mnisi, concurred: 'The best way to prevent AIDS is ABC: Abstain, Be faithful and Condomise.' Women also spoke positively abut tests for HIV antibodies, which five claimed to have taken.

A fearful rumour articulated women's concerns about potential dangers inherent in intimate biomedical interventions. Constance Zwane, a nurse at Tintswalo hospital, reportedly injected women patients with HIV on purpose. In 1996, Constance's youngest daughter, Julia, became seriously ill while studying at the University of Limpopo. Julia died from AIDS-related diseases shortly after she graduated. Women heard that Constance drew HIV-infected blood from her dying daughter's veins, kept the blood in syringes, and used it to inject patients who came to hospital for birth control injections. Constance was allegedly spiteful and did not wish Julia to die alone. Research participants claimed that she had killed several young women in this manner, and that the police had arrested her.

An adult woman believed that these stories were true. 'People don't trust Constance,' she said. 'Even if I have a cough I won't go to the hospital. I'll rather go to the [private] doctors.' But those with more intimate knowledge of the hospital's operations dismissed these allegations as fictitious. They said that new syringes come sealed from the hospital pharmacy and cannot be tampered with. Yet suspicions might have arisen because Depo-Provera, widely used as a form of birth control, is oily – almost like blood. I was also told that the police merely visited Constance's home because she was involved in a motor vehicle accident. These rumours resonate with earlier suspicions that the apartheid government had placed birth control tablets in maize meal to cause infertility among black women, and they replicate the malevolent motives of envy and revenge that are associated with witchcraft. But what is also significant to our argument is that women's critique of local health services was made from within the perspective of biomedical discourses themselves.

Men were less knowledgeable, less committed to biomedicine, and more fatalistic about the possibility that they might personally contract HIV. This orientation stemmed, in part, from their identification with 'tradition' (setšo), through which they articulated masculine interests. Boys were also less exposed to forums pervaded by public health propaganda. They disagreed with their teachers, watched football rather than soap operas on television, listened to kwaito (township hip-hop) music on the radio, hardly ever read magazines, and shied away from hospital.

The men whom I interviewed expressed confusion about HIV/AIDS. Some said that AIDS was merely 'the name that whites give mafulara' (which is associated with funeral taboos). Others described HIV/AIDS as completely new: it was 'a virus' (twatši), 'an imbalance in one's body', 'a disease of blood', or 'something to do with white blood cells'. Men were also uncertain about the transmission of HIV. Petrus Dibakwane, a temporary teacher, remarked that, during the sex act, men and women exchanged blood: after ejaculating semen, a man's penis sucked in his partner's vaginal fluids. 'I think that some men absorb too much blood from too many women. When there is too much mixture it breaks into AIDS.' Another informant was adamant that lovers could not transmit HIV if they reached orgasm at separate times. There were other misconceptions. Milton Malebe heard that, if an HIV-positive person slaughtered a cow, cut his finger, and spilt blood onto the meat, then everyone who ate that meat would be infected.

President Mbeki's controversial remarks about HIV and AIDS were a source of bemusement among men. Enios Shokane, a local political activist, told me that he had recently attended a conference of the South African Communist Party in Polokwane. Like Mbeki, the main speaker argued that a single virus cannot cause an entire syndrome. All participants then debated the issue. Enios concluded: 'We all have HIV in our blood. This is healthy. If people play it safe the virus won't cause AIDS.'

Such perceptions are not simply due to ignorance. Whereas women feared the potential misuse of biomedicine, many men actively resisted the pronouncements of public health campaigns. Daniel Shubane argued that LoveLife did not successfully combat AIDS, but merely promoted an American lifestyle. 'Look at the way they [LoveLife youth] walk and talk. You see Americans.' He was appalled by the US bombing of Afghanistan and Iraq. Other men spoke negatively about condoms. Aaron Dlamini, the former LoveLife groundbreaker, said that he thoroughly disagreed with the institution's ABC philosophy.

> This method fails. AIDS spreads at a very fast rate. I don't think this condom thing works. So many people don't use it and discourage it. With condoms, you cannot say you're safe. They can blast at any time. One man said he is allergic to the oil they put on condoms. Condoms are not natural. They are artificial … Condoms take away pleasure. They take away the real taste.

An unemployed man who had previously worked as a bank teller said defiantly, 'I never use the stuff [condoms],' and a floor polish salesman asked me: 'Why must I use condoms when I am a married man? I don't buy sex from prostitutes.' Other men speculated that the lubrication oils of condoms might contain HIV. Should one place the condoms in hot water and then in the sun, they said, one could see 'AIDS worms floating about' (McNeill 2009).[5]

In interviews, only two men admitted to having had tests for HIV antibodies. Both claimed to have tested HIV-negative. According to Enios Shokane, the ANC official, medical doctors were over-zealous in conducting these tests:

> In the hospital, they blame AIDS for every death. Long ago they did not take blood samples. Now they will test your blood – even if you only cough. Then they will tell you that you are HIV-positive and that you only have a few months to live.

Nevertheless, both women and men agreed about the sexual transmission of HIV, and allocated blame to those who engaged in unscrupulous sexual conduct. The first AIDS deaths that I recorded occurred against the backdrop of an economy of sex characterised by diverse relationships. These ranged from romantic love affairs at school, monogamous and polygamous marriages established through bridewealth transfers, informal 'take-and-sit' marriages (*vat-en-sit* in Afrikaans) and long-term extramarital liaisons (*dinyatši*) to male–male sex in the migrant compounds and in prisons, 'one-night stands' arranged in drinking houses, and purely commercial encounters with sex workers. In nearly all relations, men transferred money and gifts to their partners (Hunter 2002; Wojcicki 2002; Niehaus 2006b).

The first men who died from AIDS-related diseases were married and were among the wealthier of the poor. They were employed as labour migrants, sales representatives, drivers, teachers and policemen, and were more likely to have contracted HIV from extramarital lovers than from spouses. Lonius Mathebula, who was a teacher, allegedly contracted HIV from a colleague; Lonnet Mahlaole, a construction worker, from a paramour in Mashinini; and Sidney Manzini, a convict, from HIV-positive inmates in prison. By contrast, most women victims of AIDS were single and without stable sources of income, apart from the support of their lovers. An early victim of AIDS was Tumi Khosa, who, in a desperate attempt to support her four children after her husband's death, left Impala-hoek to seek employment in Witbank. After Tumi failed to secure a job, she started selling sex to mineworkers. She contracted HIV and returned home to die at the tender age of only 29. The other deceased women sold sexual services to long-distance truck drivers and soldiers at drinking places along the national road, or were housewives infected by their own husbands.

The allocation of blame for AIDS articulated concern about the inequalities inherent in intimate relations. Women interviewees criticised other women who went to drinking taverns late at night for contributing to the spread of HIV. But they saw masculine domination and sexual violence as ever-present nightmares that rendered them vulnerable to infection. The central villains in their discourses were therefore abusive and promiscuous boyfriends and husbands, who refused to use condoms or to test for HIV antibodies. Their comments included 'AIDS is men's fault' and 'I think my boyfriend knows about AIDS, but he pretends that it does not exist.' An archetypical story was of the husband who spent money on other women, left little cash to support his children, and infected his wife with HIV. There were also rumours of HIV-positive men who did not tell their wives of their status, and of womanisers who intentionally spread HIV by having unprotected sex with as many different partners as possible.[6]

Women research participants disputed the claim that it was men's prerogative to engage in extramarital affairs. Joyce Mathlake, who had recently separated from her boyfriend, argued fiercely that the South African government should punish promiscuous men.

We must force men above 25 to marry and say they must stay
with their wives and punish married men if we catch them with
other girls. The government must take adulterers to jail, and
married men who are out after hours.

At the same time, women complained about their financial dependence on men, and about their relative powerlessness in negotiating
safe sexual practices (Schoepf 1988: 634). Their comments included
the following: 'We women can't say, "No condom, no sex." We can't
say anything. Even if we know our husbands are fooling around. We
are male dominated. We depend upon men for our survival'; and
'Rural women should work, be economically empowered, be financially independent and be trained to run small businesses. This
reduces the time for sex.'

Male research participants described sexually promiscuous
women in unflattering terms and spoke of the dangers posed by
beautiful young women who travelled the highways, frequented
drinking houses, and were constantly on the lookout for men to
satisfy their desires for cash and commodities (Stadler 2003a).
But these stories were as much a warning as a means of allocating
blame. Some research participants recognised that women engaged
in transactional and commercial sex as a strategy for survival. As
one interviewee told me: 'Our government is the cause of AIDS. It
makes jobless women go to the streets to sell their bodies.' These
views reflect the assumption that men had sufficient autonomy to
choose their sexual partners, and sufficient authority to control the
nature of sexual encounters.

Within the household, the insinuation that a spouse was
HIV-positive was often a source of bitter conflict, and was, on at
least one occasion, the pretext for homicide. During December
2004, the chair of a local Community Police Forum (CPF) told
me of a most horrible incident that occurred in his neighbourhood.
After an extended period of absence, a man called Ferris Dube
returned to Impalahoek from his workplace in Johannesburg.
Suffering from a persistent cough, Ferris consulted a general practitioner. His wife accompanied him, and on the way back home
they quarrelled. Onlookers heard her saying that Ferris had merely
returned to Impalahoek to infect her with the 'dreaded disease'.
According to neighbours, they screamed at each other throughout
the night. The next morning smoke came from the windows of their
home. Members of the CPF broke down the door but were too
late. They discovered that Ferris had tied his wife to the bed with a

cord, dosed her with petrol, and burned her to death. He had then committed suicide by setting himself alight. Although Ferris left a note, nobody could decipher his writing.

Conspiracy theories: Dr Wouter Basson, Americans and wild beasts

Men invoked conspiracy theories that blamed forces operating well beyond local settings for the HIV/AIDS pandemic.[7] The frightening scale of the pandemic, the invisible presence of HIV within the body and official denials created an urgent need for transparency that gave conspiracy theories popular appeal (Sanders and West 2003).

The gendered nature of these theories, which were seldom embraced by women, is also significant. Conspiracy theories made greater sense to men, who were ideologically located in the public sphere, and directly encountered global institutions while working in South African cities. In blaming capricious trans-local agents for the pandemic, men articulated discontent with persistent poverty, inequality and racism. Many men were concerned that the ANC's promises of prosperity had not materialised, and that rural people remained excluded from the patrimonial politics of South Africa's new government. These discourses surfaced precisely at the time when de-industrialisation brought about the humiliating expulsion of black men from the labour force. During 1990–91, my research assistants and I conducted a social survey of 87 households in Impalahoek, and in 2003–04 we revisited all the households. Whereas the percentage of unemployed women in the sampled households remained constant, the percentage of unemployed men increased from 16 to 47 per cent. The greatest job losses occurred in mining, Pretoria's steel factories, the military, and teaching. The only increases were among taxi drivers, security guards, shop assistants, game lodge employees and farmworkers. These positions were less secure and not as well remunerated. Moreover, men did not qualify as readily as women for social security payments, such as child maintenance and foster grants.

Conspiracy theories reversed the arrow of culpability. Whereas public health and AIDS awareness discourses blamed sexually irresponsible men for spreading HIV, men's politicised discourses blamed white farmers, operatives of the former apartheid government, soldiers, undertakers and South Africa's new government for the scale of the pandemic.

During my visits to Impalahoek in 1996 and 1997, I heard persistent rumours that racist white farmers had dumped tonnes of under-grade oranges and sweet potatoes, which had been doctored with HIV, at a shopping centre and at local schools. In several homes, parents warned children that they might contract AIDS should they eat any fruit and vegetables that seemingly generous white farmers distributed in the villages. It is probable that the donation of blood oranges might have aroused suspicions. But there was also the presence of motive. Men were hard-pressed to understand why these farmers, who severely underpaid their black labourers, would suddenly give away tonnes of their produce to black people for free. One research participant, Ben Nyambi, made the following observations and raised the following questions:

> It happened here. A white farmer brought us sweet potatoes for free. I saw the truck and the white man. How could this happen? The farmer does not pay his workers well and never transports them to work. But he spent lots of money on petrol and on his truck to bring us sweet potatoes. How can he rob his workers but give us sweet potatoes for free? I think he wants to kill us.

These rumours captured constant fears that white racists might use cynical means to reduce South Africa's black population and ensure the continuation of white minority rule.[8]

Another captivating theory was that Dr Wouter Basson, the head of the former South African government's chemical weapons programme, had in fact manufactured HIV/AIDS in his laboratory, to eliminate political opponents. Many men commented on Basson's murder trial that unfolded in the South African Supreme Court during 2000. The trial brought numerous gruesome atrocities to light. It revealed that government agents planned to contaminate the drinking water of Namibian refugee camps with yellow fever and cholera germs. The security forces also dumped the bodies of 'terrorists' into the sea off the Namibian coast; gave poisoned beer to ANC operatives; and conducted experiments on the offensive use of toxins (see Chandler 2013).

For the men of Impalahoek, Dr Basson represented the archetypical evil scientist. They speculated that the apartheid government had instructed him to manufacture germs – such as those that cause cholera, but also high blood pressure and diabetes – to eliminate black people. But these genocidal plans were unsuccessful. With the help of Americans, Dr Basson therefore invented a new disease –

HIV/AIDS. In the words of research participants: 'He did research and manufactured AIDS in his laboratory. He wanted to kill people with his theory. He first tested the virus on animals and then injected humans with it'; 'It was a state chemical something, a chemical war.' Alternative suggestions were that Dr Basson merely imported HIV from the US, or that Americans had funded his research. This resonates with allegations throughout the postcolonial world that the US, where medical officials first diagnosed HIV/AIDS, was in fact the source of the virus (Farmer 1992). News reports about chemical warfare in Iraq gave added substance to these rumours.

Allegedly, Dr Basson distributed HIV by different means. He placed it in food, in water reservoirs, and in the clothes of black villagers; in the injections given to tuberculosis patients in hospitals; in smallpox vaccines; and in government-issued condoms. My research participants saw black soldiers as a prime agent for transmitting HIV. Dr Basson allegedly placed the virus in the rivers from which soldiers of the ANC's military wing, uMkhonto we Sizwe (MK), drank, and also laced the malaria tablets given to black South African Defence Force soldiers with HIV. He purposefully created a slow virus so that the soldiers could spread it to as many women as possible. But his experiments ran amok. 'Whites slept with blacks and AIDS also came to them. Now the whole world has AIDS ... This is all because of him.' Some men speculated that the court did not convict Dr Basson of murder because he alone might be able to develop a cure for AIDS. This explanation is consistent with the therapeutic principle that like combats like (Hammond-Tooke 1989: 130).

Another theory identified bestiality as the true cause of HIV and AIDS. During the early 2000s, the South African tabloid press carried regular reports of men who had sex with goats, especially in Limpopo Province (see, for example, Lubisi 2002). News reports also circulated that Taiwanese siblings in Johannesburg had punished their black domestic assistant by forcing her to have sexual intercourse with a large dog (Staff Reporter 2003). Research participants often discussed these reports and condemned these alleged acts in the strongest possible terms. Roy Mashile asked: 'How can people have sex with goats, dogs and chickens?' He exclaimed: 'This is abnormal! This is nonsense!' Roy speculated that a disorderly mixture of human and animal blood might cause HIV/AIDS. This conception resonates with Pentecostal teachings about moral depravity at the 'end of days'.

Theories of bestiality also implicated soldiers. Simon Chiloane told me that he believed that people could contract HIV only by engaging in intercourse with 'wild animals of the forest'. He suggested that HIV is in the bone marrow of baboons. Simon had heard that soldiers had had intercourse with baboons and large apes while they served on peacekeeping missions in the jungles of Rwanda and Burundi. 'Human blood mixed with animal blood causes AIDS. When the soldiers returned, they gave their wives and their girlfriends AIDS.' Another less spectacular suggestion was that diviners caused HIV/AIDS by using concoctions of baboon fat and blood to treat men's impotence.

Men also blamed South Africa's new government for doing very little to develop an AIDS vaccine. Some found it incomprehensible that AIDS was incurable and speculated that something was being concealed. Joshua Mokoena told me that a powerful Mozambican herbalist completely cured his maternal uncle (*malome*), whom doctors at Tintswalo hospital had diagnosed as HIV-positive. His uncle later returned to the hospital and was diagnosed HIV-negative. Sitting under the shade of a marula tree outside a *spaza* shop, two good friends, Dan Mokgope and Glyden Mahungela, insisted that ordinary tablets for STDs can cure AIDS. They also argued that lemon juice, squeezed onto a tampon, could absorb 'HIV germs' from a woman's vagina. Glyden was convinced that the government had already invented an AIDS cure.

> Doctors have already made an AIDS drug. They want to use it by 2005. Why not now? Why don't they make these drugs available? [He could not comprehend how nevirapine could prevent mother-to-child transmission of HIV.] How can you cure the foetus inside the womb, but not the mother?

Dan and Glyden alleged that a consortium of undertakers, coffin manufacturers, pharmaceutical corporations and surgeons, who benefited from AIDS-related deaths, had bribed powerful politicians to block the future development of an AIDS cure. These conspirators were all involved in a transnational trade in human organs. Dan and Glyden observed that some undertakers treated corpses and bereaved families with contempt. Even though black people preferred to attend funerals on Saturdays, some undertakers held them on Sundays. Undertakers were often the first to arrive on the scene of motor vehicle accidents, and there were many signs that they had tampered with corpses. Some undertakers used distant mortuaries, employed only white men to drive the hearses, and allegedly hung the corpses on hooks like slaughtered animals. One funeral parlour allowed mourners to see only the face of the deceased. 'Why? Are they afraid that you will see the whole body?' asked Glyden.

The two friends found it sinister that prominent surgeons owned mortuaries. They speculated that the surgeons secretly removed organs from the deceased, flushed out all HIV, and then shipped the organs to faraway places (such as China) for transplants. Pharmaceutical companies used the organs to manufacture drugs, and the blood bank used the deceased's blood for transfusions. Moreover, Dan and Glyden alleged that businesspeople used the organs as an ingredient in mystical potions to increase commercial profit.[9] Chinese and Indian businesspeople allegedly used human hands to entice customers to their stores. 'If you go into an Indian or a Chinese shop you smell things. You will find a very bad smell, but many people will buy at the shop. I think this is medicines mixed with the parts of dead people.' Research participants also noted that Indian traders suspiciously closed their stores for an hour each day and ceremonially washed their hands, and that Chinese traders slept in their stores overnight. Allegedly, government allowed this trade to continue because it benefited greatly from the bribes and taxes these businesspeople and corporations paid.

These theories constructed imaginative links between diseased bodies and processes in broader political and economic domains and possessed a unique aura of factuality. At the criminal trial of Dr Basson, officials of the Roodeplaat Research Laboratories testified that he had asked them to freeze-dry a small bottle of blood infected with HIV (Chandler 2013). There has also been much speculation in epidemiological literature about the prior existence of retroviruses in animal species (Hooper 1999), the South African military as a prominent route of entry for HIV (Shell 2001), and inappropriate interventions by President Mbeki's government. The appeal of these conspiracy theories, particularly to men, rests on their ideological location in the public sphere. A central theme of these theories – namely, the expendability of the poor – resonates with the experience of being made redundant from mines and industries, which operates at the heart of the South African economy. For men, conspiracy theories also provide a means to externalise blame.

Witchcraft and the reconfiguration of blame

In given situations, narratives about witchcraft, unlike those about unscrupulous sexual conduct and malevolent conspiracies, contested the very existence of AIDS. Sufferers and their kin, and the diviners and Christian healers whom they consulted, sometimes interpreted the very same complaints that physicians diagnosed as symptoms of HIV/AIDS as indices that witchcraft (*loya*) was operative.

Although witchcraft beliefs have a long and varied history in the South African lowveld, fears of bewitchment have intensified at different time periods. These included drought, population removals, and generational tensions associated with the national liberation struggle (Niehaus 2012b). Unlike the perpetrators of ritual murder, who are allegedly involved in the transnational trade of human organs, witches were insiders, such as kin and neighbours, intimately involved with their victims. Yet, at the same time, discourses of witchcraft are remarkably open-ended and allow for the constant incorporation of new themes (Geschiere 1998). Ciekawy and Geschiere argue that the witch forges a link between local kinship structures and global institutions: 'Witchcraft discourses force an opening in the village and the closed family network: after all, it is in the basic interests of the witch to betray his or her victims to outsiders' (1998: 5).

In Impalahoek, the HIV/AIDS pandemic brought about a resurgence of witchcraft accusations. Villagers did not imagine that witches could send HIV/AIDS, but they believed that witches could inflict diseases that mimicked the symptoms of AIDS. In this manner, witches took advantage of the pandemic and used it as a shield to mask their nefarious deeds (Niehaus 2013: 155–7). During 2003, Jimmy Mohale, my former research assistant, told me that he sincerely believed that many deceased persons, whom others said had suffered from AIDS-related diseases, were victims of witchcraft.

> If anybody gets ill people will say that he or she has AIDS …
> Sakkie [my nickname], I know AIDS is there! But when you die
> of AIDS your partner will also show symptoms of the disease.
> I don't think it is AIDS when a person dies, but the partner
> shows no symptoms and lives for another ten years. These cases
> are questionable.

In these questionable cases, Jimmy said, witchcraft might be operative.

Unlike in the past, accusations of witchcraft that were made in the context of the HIV/AIDS pandemic did not generate public witchhunts. Instead, the kin of the deceased secretly asked diviners to place potions called *letšwa* on the corpse. The potions allegedly made witchcraft rebound and caused the killer to die in the same manner as his or her victim. As such, mystical forms of revenge came to be used to combat mystical malevolence.

Attributions of witchcraft differed from local conspiracy theories insofar as they referred to intimate personal relations and addressed the particularities of misfortune. However, we can see both sets of discourses as responses to victim-blaming inherent in AIDS awareness propaganda. Theorists have long recognised the operation of 'projection' in discourses of witchcraft at a psychological level. Here, the subject refuses to recognise certain feelings, qualities and wishes (notably those pertaining to aggression, and, in this case, guilt); expels these from the self; and locates them in another person or thing (Kluckhohn 1944; Lambek 2002). From this perspective, we can see witchcraft as a vehicle for absolving sick persons of responsibility for their own sickness and of the blame and culpability of having infected others with a deadly virus. At the sociological level, we can also see accusations of witchcraft as bids to affect relational forms (Myhre 2009). They were attempts to counter labelling that might terminate social relations and contribute to the abjection of sick people from social networks comprising lovers, spouses, kin and neighbours. Attributions and accusations of witchcraft were bids to redraw and reconfigure social boundaries in a manner that reconnected sick persons to these networks, networks that the stigma of being HIV-positive threatened to shatter.

During fieldwork, I recorded details of 126 deaths that villagers attributed to AIDS, often by listening attentively to talk in backstage domains. In 27 of these deaths, I learned that kin and friends contested the notion that AIDS was the cause of death and claimed that witches were responsible. In 13 cases, household members accused non-kin such as neighbours, colleagues, church leaders, diviners or unnamed outsiders. This is apparent in the case of Elphas Shai, a 30-year-old man. After Elphas started working as a gardener at an electricity supply depot near Impalahoek, he developed skin lesions, experienced severe abdominal pains, and completely lost his appetite. A diviner told Elphas and his parents that an elderly woman neighbour was responsible for his sickness. The diviner alleged that she had bewitched Elphas by laying a potion called *sefolane* on the footpath he used to walk to work. The neighbour had reportedly seen Elphas carrying groceries from the supermarket to his parents and sought to eliminate him so that one of her sons could be appointed to his position. In this case, we can see the attribution of witchcraft as a bid to defend Elphas's conduct and emphasise the positive contribution he made to the household of his parents. The attribution was also a bid to reinforce the boundary between kin and non-kin, and to create solidarity within the Shai household.

In four other cases, the cognates of sick people accused their spouses or other relatives by marriage of having bewitched them. We can see these accusations as bids to cut affinal relations, constituted through the payment of bridewealth, and at the same time to strengthen ties based on consanguinity. They were also an attempt to reverse the arrow of culpability. This is apparent in the case of Moses Chiloane. Starting in 1992, when Moses lost his position as a truck driver, his wife, Lerato, supported him from the salary she earned as a teacher. Lerato bought Moses a van and gave him sufficient money to purchase beer each day. Moses contracted HIV when he cheated on Lerato with younger women. His unbecoming, reprehensible conduct provoked a great deal of unfavourable gossip throughout the neighbourhood in which he resided, particularly among Lerato's kin and colleagues. During 2002, when Moses first became severely ill, his sister alleged that Lerato had doctored him with 'love potions' (*korobela*) to win back his affection, and that the potions were now killing him. She even threw stones at Lerato's car, breaking the rear window. These allegations resurfaced after Moses died. His cognates now claimed that, when Lerato's aunt came to pray for Moses, she placed herbs underneath his mattress to hasten his death. Many outside observers did not believe that witchcraft was involved and argued that Moses' cognates were merely making these accusations to stake a claim to inheriting his estate. Yet it is highly unlikely that Moses had accumulated any savings.

A further 11 witchcraft accusations expressed intergenerational tensions, between children and parents, within the same domestic units. These accusations occurred against the backdrop of growing frustrations. Members of the younger generation committed themselves to ideologies of national liberation, which were central to the struggle against white minority rule, and to policies of development and service delivery during the post-apartheid era. In terms of these progressive temporalities (Ferguson 2006: 176–93), children anticipated that they would encounter greater status and prosperity than their parents. However, the actual experiences of young men who entered the labour market during an era of high unemployment contradicted these expectations. Sons are often quick to learn that their fathers, in fact, enjoyed greater job security, earned relatively higher wages, attained greater authority at home, and, in many cases, lived healthier and longer lives. At the same time, elders regularly blamed the younger generation for crime, sexual promiscuity and other forms of unfavourable conduct.

Young adults sometimes attributed their misfortune and relative lack of success to the witchcraft of elders. A common allegation was that, while older men worked as migrant labourers in South Africa's industrial centres, they used witch familiars, such as the snake-like *mamlambo*, to secure promotion and good salaries. But once they had retired, their witch familiars caused havoc at home and fed on the lives of their children. In these narratives, children paid with their lives for the relative success of their fathers. Jabulani Mashile retired from working in Johannesburg to take up residence with his own family in Impalahoek. Within a few years, his wife and five of his children passed away. Jabulani's remaining kin alleged that he owned a snake that killed members of his own family. However, the snake gave its victims the appearance of AIDS-like symptoms, so as not to arouse too much suspicion.

In these cases, witchcraft accusations allowed for the construction of intra-generational solidarity among the younger generation, particularly among siblings. During 2003, the sickness and death of Diana Mashile, a woman in her late twenties, provoked a great deal of discussion and debate. Diana's parents did not approve of her decision to consult diviners and they hardly ever visited her during the weeks when she stayed at a diviner's home. Diana's mother, Rhonia, reportedly told neighbours: 'I won't waste time visiting my daughter. My daughter has AIDS and she will die.' Young adults were extremely suspicious about the circumstances of Diana's death, and believed that her own parents might have been responsible. One man observed that Rhonia appeared to be proud that her daughter had AIDS. Moreover, Diana's boyfriend, Lucky, did not display any signs of sickness, and promised to contribute R300 each month towards supporting Diana's child. For this reason, my research participant argued, Diana had not died of AIDS-related diseases.

> How can Rhonia [Diana's mother] claim that she [Diana] has AIDS when her boyfriend is still alive? Jonas [Diana's father] is a Mozambican who has a snake [*mamlambo*] to feed. Rhonia loves money. They bewitch their own children so that they can get child support grants from their grandchildren. They only use AIDS as an excuse ... so that the deaths can look credible. The parents are fly-by-nights. They are witches.

In these situations, and in others, accusations of witchcraft were reactions to victim-blaming inherent in public health discourses about AIDS, and responses to the intense stigma associated with the diagnosis of being 'HIV-positive'. A significant effect of witchcraft accusations was the 'cutting of networks' (Strathern 1996: 523) and the strategic redrawing of social boundaries. Insinuations of witchcraft also created a measure of hope. Whereas persons with AIDS were destined to die, the victims of witchcraft might still be saved by diviners, who could retrieve them from their captors.

Conclusions

The allocation of responsibility, blame and culpability has been a crucial dimension of experiences of the HIV/AIDS pandemic. These processes bear important, yet also uncomfortable, implications for concepts of 'biopolitics' and 'biological citizenship'.

For some anthropologists, biomedical hegemony and a narrow focus on the somatic categories display objectivist tendencies that deflect attention from social relations and processes. In a well-known essay, Taussig (1980) argues that biomedicine tends to reify sickness by treating biological signs and symptoms as things, existing separately from the moral values, cultural meanings and social contexts in which they are embedded. He argues that in the guise of objective science, biomedicine reproduces the dominant (capitalist) political ideology and social order. Its practitioners deny any legitimacy of questions patients ask, such as 'Why me?' and 'Why now?' Taussig contrasts the narrow vision of biomedicine to the Azande theory of witchcraft, which attributes serious sickness to what he calls 'the malevolent disposition of critically relevant social relationships' (ibid.: 4). Unlike biomedicine, according to Taussig, the aetiologies of witchcraft simultaneously implicate the somatic, the physical and the moral.

The material presented in this chapter challenges the simplicity of this dichotomy. As we have seen, in Impalahoek, the allocation of blame for HIV/AIDS is the product of diverse and divergent discourses, including biomedical ones. Clinical medicine might well have objectivist tendencies. But epidemiologically informed public health interventions, such as AIDS awareness propaganda, characteristically target high-risk groups and behaviours (Balshem 1991; 1993). This tendency was most pronounced in colonial medicine, which conceptualised colonial subjects as groups, was preoccupied

by differences of race and ethnicity, and sought the cultural and
social origins of disease (Vaughan 1991). These interventions were
frequently seen as a form of victim-blaming that enhanced the stigma
of AIDS and portrayed victims as killers (at least in the era before
antiretroviral drugs). The focus on sexual infidelity accentuated
pre-existing tensions between sexual partners and contributed to
the exclusion of people with AIDS from networks of social interaction. Alternative discourses of blame – evident in malicious gossip
about malevolent nurses and conspiracy theories about agents of the
government, the military and business, as well as witchcraft accusations – exist in the same social field, alongside AIDS awareness
propaganda. They are bids to reconfigure blame and reinforce the
social relations that public health propaganda threatened to disrupt.

Not only can we contest assumptions about the objectivist
tendency of biomedicine; it is also possible to argue that the
concepts of 'biopolitics' and 'biological citizenship' underestimate the salience of non-biomedical discourses and frameworks of
perception that exist within domestic and public domains. Although
biomedical constructs have profoundly shaped the experiences of
suffering, they have not formed the basis of political mobilisation
in Impalahoek. An emphasis on the shared biological destiny of
those afflicted with HIV/AIDS detracts our attention from other,
perhaps equally salient, solidarities and divisions that are apparent
in non-biomedical discourses. Allegations about conspiracies and
witchcraft give voice to existing tensions along the lines of gender,
generation, race and class – and between village communities and
the state – that are located well beyond clinical domains.

4·
Words

During fieldwork I often heard nursing staff at Tintswalo hospital and at the Rixile HIV clinic, as well as AIDS awareness activists and home-based carers, complain that villagers shied away from undergoing voluntary counselling and testing. Yvonne Maatsie, a woman teacher who had attended several workshops on HIV/AIDS and conducted life orientation classes at school, remarked: 'People say they will die if they know [their status]. They say prevention is better than cure and for them prevention is not knowing.'

My observations and interviews in Impalahoek confirmed these impressions. During 2003 and 2004, Gunvor Jonnson and I asked the 52 research participants, selected by means of snowballing, whether they might undergo a test for HIV antibodies. Many had lost family members during the pandemic, and some personally cared for kin suffering from AIDS-related diseases. Only seven interviewees (two men and five women) claimed that they had been tested: all said that their results were negative. What struck me most was that many interviewees argued that it was better to be ignorant about one's status.

The statements by some research participants give an insight into the reasons why residents of Impalahoek were fearful, if not apprehensive, of undergoing tests for HIV antibodies. Men were usually the most outspoken. Ace Ubisi, my research assistant, whom I thought should have known better, claimed that knowledge of being HIV-positive would hasten one's death:

> Ninety-eight per cent of people from here won't go there [to test for HIV antibodies]. Only 2 per cent might go – maybe the educated ones and the Reborn Christians [*bazalwane*] ... They trust themselves. The rest of us don't. If I test HIV-positive I will die within three days. I might run away into the forest with a firearm [to commit suicide] ... If I test positive I will think all the time, thinking about dying or surviving.

Justice Kgwedi, a young man who had recently left school and was still searching for work, Jabo Nyathi, a motor mechanic, and Peter Manzini, who operated a small informal (*spaza*) trading store, expressed roughly similar views:

I hate to be tested. I hate to know that I'm going to die. I hate people telling me that I'm HIV-positive. It will be a problem because I would worry too much. When the disease and the worries get together, I will be mourning too much. I will be fighting two battles.

If someone says you are HIV-positive you won't enjoy your wife or your girlfriend. I will only check my body for TB [tuberculosis] and for other diseases – not for HIV. If you know you have HIV you will never feel alright. You will think.

I am too scared to be tested. I don't want to hear. It is all right if I die tomorrow, but it is not all right to hear I'm going to die. It will make you worry. If you are aware that you are infected, you will think too much. You will become mad.

The villagers who did test for HIV antibodies tended to do so in the latter stages of infection, and even then they tried their utmost to conceal, and avoid speaking about, their condition.

These responses differ diametrically from the 'confessional technologies' that form the cornerstone of strategies promoted by health workers and development organisations to combat HIV/ AIDS. Confessional technologies have deep social and historical roots in Europe. Born in Catholic ritual, they were redeployed with the rise of psychotherapy in the early twentieth century (Foucault 1980). The notion of the 'talking cure' also characterises 'coming out' narratives that have emerged among gay communities within the US since the 1960s. Here, acceptance and liberation were to be found in bringing one's innermost, authentic self to words (Weston 1997: 44–51). Ideologies of religious salvation, psychoanalysis and sexual liberation all inform public health interventions in the HIV/AIDS pandemic.[1] In the context of HIV/AIDS, confessional technologies comprise voluntary counselling and testing (VCT), 'coming out' with HIV positivity, and providing public testimony about sickness and the positive transformative effects of medication (Nguyen 2009; 2010).

According to Nguyen (2005: 131), confessional technologies 'have proven robust even in the alien soil of an impoverished Africa'. He shows how, in West African cities, 'talking groups' flourished among AIDS awareness activists. The groups adopted self-disclosure as a means of fashioning the self, forging social solidarity, and accessing treatment and other resources (ibid.). In South Africa, too, VCT has formed the basis of medical interventions in the case of HIV/AIDS. Activists of the urban-based Treatment Action Campaign (TAC) have been the most vociferous proponents of 'confessional technologies'. Led by the world-renowned civil and gay rights activist Zackie Achmat, they have used disclosure as a means of creating a new identity, and have deployed storytelling as a means of personal and collective empowerment. Throughout the country, expensive billboards promoting the LoveLife campaign simply proclaim 'Talk!'

But not all South Africans have embraced these cosmopolitan technologies. My research participants were by no means alone in their choice not to ascertain their HIV status. During the mid-1990s, researchers offered 2,500 residents in the mining town of Carletonville free and anonymous tests for HIV antibodies. Not a single person accepted (Ashforth 2002: 122). A random survey from the same period found that only 58 (8 per cent) of 726 HIV-positive patients had told others of their status (Pawninski and Lalloo 2001: 448). People's refusal to test is partly, but not completely, due to the lack of treatment options. The Anglo American mining corporation offered free antiretroviral treatment to its employees well before the public sector roll-out of antiretroviral drugs. Yet, by 2005, only 7,348 (22 per cent) of an estimated 33,500 HIV-positive employees had enrolled in the company's wellness programme (George 2006: 185–6).

During the post-Mbeki era, successive campaigns by South Africa's Health Ministry to promote testing have generated some improvement. A National Communications Survey found that, by 2009, 32 per cent of men and 71 per cent of women had tested for HIV antibodies (Government of South Africa 2010).[2] But such figures might well be over-optimistic. People at high risk of HIV infection, such as victims of gender-based violence, were not more likely to get tested (Steven et al. 2010). Moreover, testing by itself does not guarantee the anticipated benefits. During an AIDS awareness campaign at the University of Limpopo, 17 per cent of first-year students underwent VCT, but only 20 per cent of these students came for their results (Oxlund 2009: 225).

In this chapter, I seek to unravel the complex social reasons and cultural logic that inform people's choice to remain ignorant about their HIV status, which might well constitute a 'hidden form of resistance' (Scott 1990) to health propaganda. In this respect, I aim to build on previous studies by Stadler (2003b), Wood and Lambert (2008) and McNeill (2011), who examine silence, secrecy and coded talk as responses to HIV/AIDS in various parts of South Africa's rural periphery. It stands to reason, given the ethnographic evidence presented in the previous two chapters, that the decision not to test for HIV antibodies might constitute an attempt to avoid the imposition of a stigmatised identity, and, perhaps more importantly, to avoid confronting culpability for the deaths of former sexual partners. But, in addition to these pragmatic concerns, I contend that the strategies of silence and secrecy are informed by assumptions about the intrinsic power and the transformative capacity of words. I suggest that, while AIDS awareness activists, such as members of the TAC, embrace the potential of speech to liberate, residents of Impalahoek fear the potentially dangerous impact of words, as in being pronounced 'HIV-positive'. I argue that such words can be perceived as deadly. In local knowledge, they crystallise sickness, invoke negative emotions associated with pending death, and thereby worsen suffering.

'If I test HIV-positive I will die'

One cannot ascribe people's disinclination to test for HIV antibodies to the absence of exposure to biomedical knowledge. As we have seen, public healthcare initiatives and popular discourses have ensured a super-abundance of information. My research participants tended to over- rather than underestimate the prevalence and contagiousness of HIV and the deadliness of AIDS.

Even seasoned health workers, such as Aaron Dlamini, who worked as a groundbreaker at the LoveLife Y-Centre and taught teenagers to live a positive lifestyle in the context of the pandemic, was reluctant to test for HIV antibodies. Aaron's words echoed the views of others:

> I have never heard of a single person going for an HIV test ...
> When they tell you, you automatically become a living dead. If
> you talk about it, it becomes worse. In this way, they [possibly
> nurses and neighbours] put a negative stigma on you. If you
> know [your status] you will survive one year; if you don't know
> it may even be five or ten years. You worry, and you worry that
> you worry. You worry twice. You will think, and you will dream
> of a grave all the time. In your mind you will see death and what
> happens to your body.

A more plausible explanation than ignorance might be a fatalistic acceptance of one's destiny in the absence of alternative treatment options. Prior to the public-sector roll-out of HAART, biomedical practitioners were capable merely of treating the symptoms of AIDS-related diseases, and hospital amenities, particularly in the tuberculosis ward, were spartan. But even under these conditions, there were clear advantages of knowing one's HIV status. People who had tested 'negative' could put their minds at rest, while those who had tested 'positive' could at least protect their sexual partners and breastfed babies from being infected with a potentially deadly virus. They could also protect themselves from re-infection. In addition, even in the initial stages of the pandemic, an HIV-positive diagnosis was a prerequisite to securing social grants – a highly valued and significant source of income, particularly in poorer households.[3]

Another significant factor might be the fear of social stigma, as evident in the perception of HIV-positive persons as 'dead before dying', and the recognition of culpability for having infected past and present sexual partners with a potentially deadly virus (McNeill and Niehaus 2009: 33–9). But the relationship between testing HIV-positive and shame was not nearly as direct as one might suppose. People could simply undertake an HIV test elsewhere and conceal their status from kin and neighbours. Refusing to undertake a test was also no guarantee of avoiding discrimination and social ostracism. It was extremely hard to conceal the symptoms of AIDS, which were well known throughout Bushbuckridge. Constant coughing, drastic weight loss, ugly skin lesions and fluffy hair were sufficient in themselves to provoke prejudice and generate the most malicious forms of gossip.

Since 2005, the availability of HAART at Rixile clinic has drastically improved treatment options. Clinical evidence shows eminently reasonable rates of retention among people initiated on treatment at the clinic (MacPherson et al. 2008). In this context, HAART has enhanced the chances of HIV-positive persons living full and productive lives. These changes have weakened the association between AIDS and death and have consequently also eroded the fears of testing HIV-positive. But many sick people are still reluctant to report to medical facilities and saw testing for HIV antibodies as a 'last resort'.[4]

A careful re-examination of the statements by interviewees suggests that they do not simply fear knowing that they suffer from an incurable, potentially fatal, condition. My research participants were petrified of hearing medical personnel and others pronounce that they were 'HIV-positive'. This is apparent in the following statements by men, cited in the opening section of this chapter: 'I hate people *telling* me that I'm HIV-positive'; 'If someone *says* you are HIV-positive'; 'I don't want to *hear*'; and 'When they *tell* you'.

My research participants seemed to be less concerned that neighbours might see their condition than they were about the prospect that neighbours might speak about it. Aaron Dlamini, the former AIDS educationist, said that he would be furious if anyone ever said his brother had AIDS. 'Even if he is correct, I will beat him.' Lissie Mohlala, a secretarial worker at the Bushbuckridge municipality, responded as follows when I asked her whether she had tested for HIV antibodies:

> I might go [for testing], but I will definitely not go around here. There are many people here and they gossip, especially the nurses and your friends. They are the ones who gossip the most. The nurses will tell you that you have AIDS and they will tell you what your CD4 count is. But they will also tell your friends, show them the pills and gossip about you. If you know you are HIV-positive you will have stress. You will ignore to eat, and you will be unable to sleep. You will die. You will always think about death.

Aaron's and Lissie's statements express a belief that speech itself could be deadly, and that words themselves might possess intrinsic agency and transformative power (Basso 1969). Words such as 'HIV' and 'AIDS' seem to have the capacity to bring to consciousness and materialise the status of persons as being afflicted with death.

The fear of powerful words was not merely evident in people's reluctance to speak about HIV/AIDS in public domains. In Impalahoek, as indeed elsewhere in South Africa, talk about AIDS was confined to backstage regions of social interaction (Stadler 2003b; McNeill and Niehaus 2009: 60–5). Moreover, even when speaking about the third person in contexts of gossip, people avoided mentioning the words 'HIV' and 'AIDS' directly (Wood and Lambert 2008). Research participants suggested that it was not simply impolite to mention these words: their articulation might have very dangerous consequences.[5] Instead, they deployed a broad range of creative euphemisms. Villagers would say that an infected person suffered from the 'three letters' (*maina a mararo*), 'germs' (*twatši*), 'the painful sickness' (*kukuana hloko*), or from 'the fashionable disease' (*bolwetši gona bjalo*); that they had purchased 'a single ticket' (in English), were on a 'diet' (*dayeta*), or had 'eaten herbs that make one disappear' (*enga moragela kgole*). My research assistants and I soon learned to refer to HIV/AIDS as 'the dreaded disease' during fieldwork and in interviews.

The agency of words

The notion that words possess intrinsic agency was seldom formulated explicitly. But it could be inferred from several observations, in
contexts that initially seemed to me to have little to do with sickness
and healing.

On a Saturday in 2005 I took a break from fieldwork to visit the
Mount Sheba Nature Reserve with research assistants from Impalahoek. My friends were struck by the exceptional beauty of nature.
Ace Ubisi, who was once an active church-goer, said that he found
it incomprehensible that God could have created the mountains,
valleys and forests in only six days. 'It took 200 men two years to
build the new police station and jail in Impalahoek, so how could
God make all of this in only six days,' he asked. Ace's maternal uncle,
who was a preacher of the Zion Christian Church (ZCC), tried to
eliminate Ace's confusion. God, he said, brought nature into being
through the act of divine speech. 'In the Bible we read that God
would say "Let there be light!" and the light appeared. He would
also say "Let there be mountains and waters!" and the mountains
and waters appeared.' Christian cosmology equates the very act of
creation with divine speech.

A belief in the power of words was also apparent in secular contexts.
In 1996, South Africa's national football team, Bafana Bafana,
participated in the World Cup tournament in France. I watched the
opening game between South Africa and the host nation with friends
in Impalahoek. I did not entertain high hopes. Bafana Bafana fielded
an inexperienced team that had never come close to beating top
opposition sides. But, to my surprise, everyone else told me that they
expected Bafana Bafana to win – not merely the game, but also the
tournament. Some predicted that the final would be against Nigeria,
another popular African team. I was astonished. My friends included
football coaches, an accomplished referee, and a former player in
South Africa's Premier League – who knew far more about the game
than I did. Bafana Bafana lost the opening game 0–3 to France and
suffered the humiliation of being eliminated after the first round of
the tournament. Only much later did some of my friends admit that
they, too, expected South Africa to lose, but they could not bring
themselves to say so. As an avid football fan explained to me: 'If you
say South Africa will lose, we will lose. When we played Switzerland,
all South Africans said we would win and we won.'

Words seem to possess a certain materiality, and were on occasion treated as if they were things. My research assistants and I were

eager to learn about a certain episode of witchcraft accusation. We heard that, after several instances of misfortune had occurred at a local bakery, all employees hired a bus to consult a witch-diviner close to the Swaziland border. The diviner apparently revealed three witches among the bakery employees. We approached several potential informants, but they all referred us to the shop steward, Freddy Malene. Freddy had organised the witch-hunt and, for this reason, his employers had suspended him from work. Freddy warmly welcomed us and offered a very detailed account of events at the bakery. At the end of the interview, we briefly gave Freddy advice, saying that his employer could not dismiss him without proper warning, and urging him to consult the legal advisers of his trade union. Freddy's mother overheard our conversation and, as we were about to leave, thanked us 'for the words you gave my son'. To express her gratitude, she offered me a beautiful reed mat, which must have taken her a week to manufacture. I accepted the mat, although I eventually paid for it. But I left thinking: are words so concrete that they can be reciprocated with gifts?

In Impalahoek, one could observe the constructive power of speech during invocations to the ancestors, Christian hymns, prayers and confessions. Whenever some men set off to seek work in Johannesburg, they would call their paternal aunt (*rakgadi*) and kneel with her at an isolated spot in the yard. She would then sip a maize drink and spit the liquid in all four directions, proclaiming: 'Fathers. Here is Fundani! He is going to work in Johannesburg! Give him luck! Let him get work!' Migrants labourers also invoked the ancestors upon returning from work and would then thank them for their protection and support.[6]

In the numerous Zionist, Apostolic and Pentecostal churches of Impalahoek, prayers were seldom silent. During sermons and prayer meetings, congregants were expected to kneel on the ground and to pray loudly to God, as if screaming out the words. Their individual voices mingled in a cacophony of sound (Comaroff 1985: 245–7). Believers widely acknowledged the miraculous power of prayer. Father Ngobeni, who was a wealthy storeowner and founder of the Pentecostal Crusade, reportedly prayed earnestly after thieves stole from his store. Within days, the thieves came to him to ask for forgiveness and returned all the cash and belongings that they had taken. Some local churches occasionally deployed confession (*ipolela*) as a means of managing the moral conduct of their congregants. I never confessed myself, but I did observe Zionist church members meeting with ministers out of earshot of the congregation. One confessant told me that he had engaged in a romantic extramarital affair and afterwards suffered remorse (*pona molato*; literally, 'seeing problems in oneself'). After verbalising what he had done, the minister simply replied: 'This is sin! May God forgive you!' 'Hereafter I immediately felt relief,' he told me. Unlike prayer, confessions were strictly private.

Deadly words, unfortunate names, and curses

As shown, residents of Impalahoek acknowledged the agency of words, and, in certain contexts, ranging from sport to religion, they deployed speech in a constructive manner. These meanings might well support 'confessional technologies', as employed by activists of the TAC, as a means of confronting HIV and AIDS (Nguyen 2009; Robins 2006). But there seems to be one crucial difference: in Impalahoek, fear of the dangerous and destructive potential of words seems to outweigh faith in their therapeutic potential. This, too, was apparent in numerous everyday contexts.

Gossip and swearing provoked severe unease among research participants. Jonsson (2004: 23) writes that young women in Impalahoek very seldom discussed sex or private affairs with each other, and when they did talk about these topics, they generally spoke in the third person. Young women distrusted each other and feared that gossip might spoil their reputations. One good thing about having boyfriends, they said, was that they could talk with them about intimate matters without provoking envy. People took even greater offence at swear words, particularly when others insulted their mothers. Men who swore frequently used the Afrikaans words *bliksem* ('lightning') and *moerskont* (literally 'mother's vagina') as if they were acting outside themselves and dissociating themselves from the spoken words. (Vernacular terms were generally deemed to be more powerful.) Others swore by calling people animal names. I heard a woman shout 'donkey' (*bongolo*) and 'witch familiar' (*thuri*) at her disobedient daughter when she was in a state of rage.

Certain words, which were not necessarily swear words, seemed to have the power to disrupt social hierarchy, create envy and conflict, provoke disgust, and unleash powerful emotions. Rules of respect (*hlonipa*) dictated that it was morally inappropriate to pronounce such words in certain social contexts. For example, younger persons were not allowed to call elders by name; they had to address related elders by kinship terms such as 'maternal uncle' (*malome*), and unrelated adults by their relation to their peers, such as 'mother of

Fundani' (*MmaFundani*). Nor were younger persons allowed to ask elders where they had been, since the answer might prove embarrassing. They were not allowed to say directly that an elder was drunk, but instead had to use the euphemisms 'he chases goats' (*o kgapa diputi*) or 'he has eaten maize' (*a jele mabele*). Villagers also had to deploy euphemisms when referring to urination or excretion. Instead of saying 'urinate' (*rota*), villagers had to use the phrases 'blindfold rats' (*fahla magotla*) or 'spill water' (*ntšha meetse*). Instead of 'excrete' (*nya*), they had to say 'I'm going outside' (*go ya ntla*) or 'I'm going to send myself' (*ke nyaka go te thoma*).

As we have seen, talk about sex and death was strictly proscribed. A male teacher told me that he found it exceptionally difficult to teach sex education as part of the curriculum for life orientation. In local convention, he said, it was taboo to refer to sexual organs when addressing children. Instead, he decided to use the English alternatives. 'Had I used the Northern Sotho terms, their parents might even have demanded my resignation,' the teacher explained to me. Notable exceptions were the mother's brother and father's younger siblings, who could speak to younger people about sex in a pedagogical manner. Moreover, grandparents, who were of a different generation, could tease grandchildren about sexual matters, and cross-cousins, who had a joking relationship with each other, shared lewd humour. But the most intimate forms of talk about sex occurred between spouses, lovers, coevals and friends, and also with outsiders, such as anthropologists, who were of the same generation. But even in the latter contexts, people frequently employed euphemisms for sexual intercourse.

To avoid unleashing strong negative emotions, villagers avoided direct reference to death. In many contexts, adults signified death by non-verbal means. For example, an initiation master indicated that a young man had died at a circumcision lodge by breaking a clay pot in front of his mother.[7] Symbolic inversions, such as turning around logs in a fire and placing their thick ends in the centre, also signified death (Berglund 1976: 230–8).

Common euphemisms for death were that the deceased had been 'taken by a hyena' (*tšerwe ke Phiri/ditau*) or 'gone to the place of the ancestors' (*o ile badimong*); that they had 'rested' (*o e thobalatetše*); or that the 'house has fallen' (*o wetše ke ntlo*), the 'water had dried up' (*meetse a pshele*) or the 'sun had set' (*dikeletswe ke letšatsi*).

Research participants were sensitive to the dissonance between words and their empirical referents. I often cross-checked the information supplied to me and I was surprised how seldom people lied.

Men and women shied away from unpleasant facts through omission, and by distorting minor details in the story. But they hardly ever invented facts. They were usually honest, sometimes brutally so. A former prisoner told me that he was officially incarcerated for the 'illegal possession of a firearm'. But, he said, the police should have arrested him for 'attempted murder'. The firearm belonged to a man who had hired him to kill his wife's lover, but friends of his intended victim overpowered him before he could shoot. For my research participant, it was more important to tell the truth than portray himself in a positive light.

This concern seems to relate to broader anxieties about the predictive power of words. In Impalahoek, and throughout the South Africa lowveld, there has been hardly any tradition of prophecy. People seem to fear that the pronouncement of unpleasant words might bring about unpleasant consequences. Mabetha Monareng recalled that, during 1986, lightning struck next to a Zionist church, killing two boys and two cows. Neighbours incorrectly informed Mabetha's mother that he was one of the deceased. When Mabetha arrived home, his mother was overjoyed to see that he was still alive. But she immediately placed ash, a cooling substance, on Mabetha's forehead, to protect him against the destructive power of the pronouncement.

Personal names, too, were deemed to possess special agency. In Impalahoek, individuals had up to six different names. Whereas mothers gave birth to babies, fathers named them and bestowed them with social identity. A baby's first name usually pertained to an incident that occurred at the time of his or her birth. For example, a man named his son Soweto because he was visiting this city at the time of the baby's birth. Children soon earned additional names. Nurses and teachers conferred on them English or Afrikaans names, which they subsequently used when interacting with white employers and government bureaucracies. Such names were often taken from the Bible. The third name was generally that of an ancestor. Elders sometimes interpreted a baby's incessant crying as a sign that a forgotten ancestor was plaguing him or her. The crying, they believed, would stop only once a diviner had identified the responsible ancestor and parents appeased the ancestor by naming the baby after him or her (Mönnig 1983: 102–7). Children also earned nicknames (*dikwero*) from their playmates and peers. These could include Lepara (walking stick), Badzy (cousin), Duma (noisy or talkative), or Dubuka (a helpful person). Finally, upon returning home from the circumcision lodge, a boy was entitled to give himself his own name. Kelebotse ('I am handsome') is an appropriate example.

Research participants were adamant that names were not simply rhetorical but described a person's character and disposition. It was never quite clear whether the character or disposition led to the name or vice versa. Naming a person after an ancestor created a special bond. One man was named after his maternal great-grandmother, called Ramadimabe ('father of misfortune'). He explained that she was prone to misfortune, but also extremely resilient and able to contain the misfortune she experienced. 'Like her,' he said, 'my life has also been a life of long suffering, but I am also resilient and tough.' Other informants, too, told me that they appropriated the dispositions of the ancestors after whom they were named. Mbhekeni said that, like his great-grandfather, he tended to be short-tempered. Kotšo (derived from the Northern Sotho word for 'peace', kgotšo) told me that, like his great-grandfather, he was rude and fortunate in money matters. In ritual contexts, a person named after the most senior ancestor was treated as the most senior sibling, even though he or she might not actually be the first-born.

Names that referred to specific events at the time of a person's birth could also shape his or her destiny. A woman named Bareforiye ('we have been calmed') claimed that she was good at resolving disputes. Mohlopeng ('someone who is troubled') told me that, as a child, he was always restless and cried throughout the night. As he grew older, he was prone to bouts of aggression. Lekhudani ('one who is ill') said, 'Even as an adult I have never been well.' Tshiki-wane ('to be abandoned') was forsaken by her own parents, and later deserted by her husband. 'I believe you follow your name,' she told me. 'What I have lived throughout my life was the same as my name.' In these instances, it was deemed impossible to avoid one's destiny. This is captured by the saying 'Tolerate a good name; tolerate a bad name' (Lebitso lelebotse seroma; lebitso lebe seroma).

Anxiety about the potential destructive agency of words was most apparent in witchcraft. Anthropological researchers have noted that, whereas Mediterranean people tend to fear the malevolent power of sight, as in the evil eye (Galt 1982), in much of Southern Africa people fear the malevolent power of sound, as in curses.[8] West (2007) observes that Muedans in Mozambique construct sorcery through speech and experience it through threats and accusations. 'People do not speak of sorcery', he writes, 'they actually speak sorcery' (ibid.: 21). The material I collected in Impalahoek, located on the opposite side of the Mozambique–South Africa border, confirms some of these observations. It would be unwise to reduce witchcraft to words, only because these words often have very real material referents, such as concrete episodes of misfortune. But, nonetheless, the power of cursing was apparent in numerous examples. The most well-known curse was the simple expression 'I'll see you!' (*Ke tlo go bona!*). These words were purported to have deadly consequences, particularly when the speaker possessed innate malevolent power.

Two incidents that were widely discussed in Impalahoek attest to the destructive power of cursing. The first concerned Rexon Khoza, who suspected another man of engaging in an extramarital love affair with his wife. Rexon confronted this man in public and, in a state of rage, screamed at him: 'I'll see you.' Only two days later, an unknown assailant shot dead his wife's lover in what appeared to be a robbery. Some neighbours were convinced that Rexon harboured the power of witchcraft. Others insisted that the lover's death was coincidental. The second incident pertained to Khazamula Nyathi, a man in his seventies who was the leader of the local *muchongolo* dance team (Niehaus and Stadler 2004). At one gathering, Khazamula's 28-year-old grandson, Maguduza Nyathi, a lawyer, said that he would never dance for the team. A fierce argument erupted. Khazamula apparently shouted at Maguduza, 'You are a Shangaan! *Muchongolo* is our tradition!' He then beat him with a stick. Maguduza retaliated and beat his grandfather with his fists. Then, Khazamula reportedly cursed him, saying: 'For beating me, you'll die! You think I'm nothing and that you're a lawyer. I'm your grandfather. You can be a lawyer in heaven or in hell.' Just one month later, Maguduza tried to separate two fighting men at a drinking tavern and was fatally wounded. Onlookers believed that Khazamula's curse was the 'second spear' (Evans-Pritchard 1937: 26) that had brought about his death.

In a practice referred to as 'bottling', football players used words in a destructive manner. Ace Ubisi, who was a striker for Impalahoek Fast Eleven during the late 1980s, recalled that their team manager sometimes brought a bottle containing strong, dark-coloured potions that smelled like rum to the team's camp. Three hours before the game, the manager would ask Ace to speak the name of his opponent into the bottle. Ace recalled that he usually said words such as: 'Givens! My name is Ace! I'm going to play against you. Today I bottle you! You have nowhere to go!' Ace then breathed into the bottle. The manager would then close the lid and bury the bottle in a termite hill,[9] about ten metres behind the penalty box. Ace sincerely believed that bottling rendered opposition defenders useless on match days. Players defended the legitimacy of this practice by saying that, unlike witchcraft, which was meant to kill, the bottling of football players merely ensured victory.

Powerful words were also deployed as vengeance magic (*letšwa*) to make witchcraft rebound. Loicy Shai told me that she once suspected that she might have been a victim of witchcraft. She was unable to find work, her fiancé left her for another woman, and she was plagued by the most horrible nightmares: for example, she would dream that her younger sister, who was still alive, was deceased. A Zionist healer revealed to Loicy that her former boyfriend's mother had spoken a curse against her. The healer instructed Loicy to do the following. She had to take a Coca-Cola bottle, verbalise her distress and anger by speaking into it, and immediately close its lid. She then had to take the bottle to a crossroads, smash it on a stone, and walk away without looking back. 'This,' the healer said, 'will remove your misfortune [*bati*]. It will cause those who want you to suffer to suffer.' Within a year after Loicy had performed the ritual, she secured a secretarial position at the Bushbuckridge municipality and found a new boyfriend.

Sickness, silence and discreet speech

This rather lengthy discussion of beliefs regarding the potential agency of words serves as a necessary backdrop for understanding why men and women should display intense fear at hearing medical personnel pronounce that they had tested 'HIV-positive'. In local knowledge, such a statement had the same destructive capacity as a curse that might materialise sickness and death. Anxiety about the potential effects of deadly words also illuminates the tendency among local residents to avoid mentioning 'HIV' and 'AIDS', particularly in public domains of interaction. Unlike activists of the urban-based TAC, residents of Impalahoek have not deployed 'confessional technologies' to confront the pandemic (Nguyen 2009), but have creatively used concealment and silence, and on occasion also indirect and discreet speech.

Klaits' (2010) analysis of the logic of speech in an Apostolic church in Botswana provides some insight into reasons for the prominence of silence and discreet speech in Impalahoek. He observes that church members perceived faith (*tumelo*) as being vital to healing. In cases of sickness, they communicated faith and love from their own bodies to those of persons who were unwell. For church members, hymns, prayers and words of compassion not only mitigated harm but also assisted healing. By the same token, expressions of scorn and envy were morally inappropriate forms of speech that worsened suffering. The church members avoided certain topics. To protect themselves from the power of witchcraft, they refrained from thinking and speaking about it.

Klaits' argument, which builds on earlier observations on the public sphere in Botswana (Durham and Klaits 2002), suggests a broader perspective on therapeutic interventions, one that recognises the significance of words in the creation of social affect and in healing. Carers were expected to comfort and strengthen (*phorola*) the sick person verbally, and thereby create hope and faith in recovery, even if these expectations might seem to be unrealistic. In this context, it was understandable and completely acceptable to tell white lies. Conny Nyathi, a home-based carer, told me: 'If you wish a person must live you must rejuvenate him with words, with words from the mouth. You must promise them they will live.' She recalled visiting a terminally ill man who told her that he was extremely depressed that his wife had abandoned him when he most needed her help. 'Do not worry!' Conny told him. 'When you have recovered, and you are no longer ill, she will return.' A Wesleyan minister regularly accompanied members of his small congregation to pray for seriously ill persons (who might well be afflicted with AIDS-related diseases). The Methodists did not enter the room but stood in the yard, praying aloud and singing hymns, so that the sick person could hear their words. 'We show that we love them. We say nothing about their condition. We only say that we believe God will save them.' The minister did not specify whether he referred to physical or spiritual salvation.

Conversely, it was deemed improper for carers and others to speak about any topic that might upset the sick person. They were not expected to name his or her illness, especially not when their condition was grave. MacBeth Shai, a middle-aged teacher, observed that elderly members of his family were sometimes reluctant to attend hospital when ill, precisely because they feared that the nursing staff might 'use negative words'. 'The nurses would say that they are too old, and that they are in hospital crying for help.' He observed that diviners were always more positive. Although diviners might say that a client's condition was 'terrible', they would always promise recovery. 'The diviners say we need to work hard and do one, two and three.'

During fieldwork, I consulted Dr Van Heerden, an Afrikaans-speaking private general practitioner, about a medical problem.

I spoke very positively about his services to research participants. For only a small fee, he had made an excellent diagnosis, and had effectively performed minor surgery on me in his consulting room. I also relayed that Dr Van Heerden had admonished me about my diet and lack of exercise. To my surprise, my research participants criticised the directness of his speech to me and observed that locally the doctor had a very unsavoury reputation on account of the unkind words he spoke.

Anyone who announced that a sick person had been diagnosed HIV-positive, or as suffering from AIDS-related diseases, conveyed the impression that he or she might wish for the sick person to die. Givens Thobela recalled the great sensitivity with which his grandmother spoke about the medical condition of his maternal uncle (*malome*). Givens' uncle was struck down by illness while working as a farm labourer; he was taken to hospital and eventually became bedridden at home. His grandmother grouped together all the younger members of the Thobela family and told them: 'We have different diseases. There is tuberculosis and gonorrhoea [*toropo*]. Your uncle does not have these diseases. He has the disease of today [*ke bolwetši bja gona bjalo*].' Givens compared discreet speech to a book. 'You cannot judge a book by its cover,' he said. 'You have to open the book and read it. We could see that my maternal uncle had flying [fluffy] hair, coughed blood and was unable to walk.'

Women volunteers who provided home-based care for people living with AIDS had learned to work with great discretion and to maintain the utmost confidentiality. Nurses at Tintswalo hospital issued the carers with medical cards, providing a profile of the patient's treatment history. The cards never explicitly indicated that a patient had tested positive for HIV antibodies. One home-based carer explained:

> Sometimes, on the corner of the card, there would be a picture of a book. This tells us that the person has AIDS. You must never say it out loud. The patients usually conceal this. Even the family members may not know.

Villagers condemned those who spoke too freely about AIDS. On a few occasions, indiscreet speech had provoked accusations of witchcraft (see Chapter 3). Jabo Malale, a young man, told me how incensed he was when an elderly neighbour told him that his terminally ill mother 'might die before month-end'. The neighbour also gossiped to her friends, saying that Jabo's mother might have to be cremated by the government because her children were too poor to afford a coffin. 'She was very impolite,' Jabo told me. 'Those words are evil.' He suspected that the neighbour had bewitched his mother: she was allegedly envious because Jabo had bought his mother groceries when he was employed, while the neighbour's own children used their wages to purchase liquor. Kin and carers secluded terminally sick people, not only to protect them from the physical pollution, but also to preclude outsiders from speaking about their condition.

Silence and discreet speech were also required at funerals. In Botswana, Durham and Klaits (2002) and Klaits (2009) observed that attendees at funerals sought to participate in the well-being and suffering of others. Through supportive words, prayers and hymns they disclosed sympathetic concern that militated against the harm that would otherwise be caused. This was particularly the case during the night vigil, when attendees sought to comfort and strengthen the bereaved family for the ensuing events. During the actual funeral service, which was held in the yard or church hall the next morning, different speakers represented the therapy management group and distinct categories of kin, as well as the professional bodies, organisations and churches to which the deceased belonged. There were further prayers and hymns at the graveyard, and speeches by the funeral undertakers, headman and municipal councillor to thank the mourners. Speakers selectively emphasised the positive aspects of the deceased's life and works, and carefully edited out, or concealed, less palatable aspects of his or her biography. In many cases they purposefully constructed a contrived reality, and at times portrayed notorious gangsters as honourable church-goers. They did this, I was told, so as not to offend the aura (*seriti*) or breath (*moya*) of the deceased (see Niehaus 2013: 189).

At funerals, a specific orator was chosen to provide a speech about the cause of death. He or she usually spoke in the vaguest and most cryptic of terms. For example, the orator might say that the deceased had suffered from a 'long' or 'short' sickness. My inquiries as to the cause of death provoked quite unexpected answers. At times, kin and neighbours remarked that the deceased had complained of a 'headache' or even 'tooth pain' before he or she had passed away. Further prompting elicited the response that doctors failed to relay the nature of the sickness to kin, or even the put-down 'we do not talk about these things'. It was deemed highly improper to say that someone had died from AIDS-related diseases. Not only would this cast aspersions on his or her character (Wood and Lambert 2008:

226), but it would also prophesise the imminent death of surviving spouses and sexual partners. A preacher of the ZCC, who attended up to four funerals each month, told me that he had never heard a single person speak about HIV/AIDS. 'Rumours might fly about, but people [presumably the orators] do not announce it.' The Wesleyan minister said that, although he sometimes addressed congregants about AIDS at the church hall, he explicitly advised pastors not to say anything about AIDS at funerals.

> It is not necessary. We only come to comfort people. Should I speak about AIDS, the family might hit me. They would say that I am not a doctor. This would be an abomination to people. For them it would be very shameful.

Since 2005, the availability of HAART had drastically improved the prospects of persons infected with HIV and has the potential to transform AIDS from a terminal sickness to a chronic, manageable, condition. The gradual uncoupling of HIV/AIDS and death has lessened people's reluctance to test for HIV antibodies and speak about their condition. My research participants still perceived AIDS as a life-threatening and stigmatising condition, and feared hearing medical personnel pronounce that they were 'HIV-positive'. Sick people often delayed testing until they were severely ill and, as a consequence, late presentation and advanced levels of immuno-suppression were formidable barriers to effective treatment (Mfecane 2011; MacPherson et al. 2008: 590).

HAART did not generate a spate of confessions. Yet, people who attended support group meetings at Rixile clinic, used HAART, and had witnessed some improvement in their condition began discreetly telling outsiders about their health. The pronouncement was not that their status was 'HIV-positive', but rather that they were 'using tablets' (a euphemism for receiving HAART). Only in 2007 did I hear a person confess to living with HIV/AIDS. While consuming chicken and maize porridge at a local eatery, a man asked my research assistants, with whom he was well acquainted, whether they wanted his soft drink. 'These days I am not so well,' he said. 'My appetite is poor. I'm going to Rixile for tablets.' We were all surprised by his openness. Subsequently, we heard of AIDS activists such as May Mokoena who were addressing different constituencies such as teachers about his experiences of sickness and recovery. Like May, ordinary persons infected with HIV spoke about their condition only when receiving effective medication. But unlike him, they would only tell those whom they trusted. One research participant, a general labourer at the Bushbuckridge municipality, recalled that he met Lakios Malatsi, a colleague, standing outside a drinking tavern. Lakios told the research participant that his wife had infected him with HIV, but that he still loved her, and that, together, they were now being treated at Rixile clinic. Lakios wanted to confront his wife's extramarital lover and tell him that she was HIV-positive, but he did not wish to do so in front of any other people.

Much supportive talk advertised the positive effects of HAART. Custom Chiloane relayed to me that his friend, Lucas Malebe, who was seriously ill, had lost all hope of recovery, and refused to go to hospital. Custom was shocked because he had anticipated a more positive response from his friend.

> Lucas told me, 'There is no need for me to go to hospital. I will go there, I will return, and I'll still be sick. No doctor or nurse can help me. The best thing is simply to stay here and die. I was involved with three girls. They all died. People gossiped that it was HIV.'
>
> Lucas lay in bed waiting for death. I think his problem was hope. I went home and came up with a strategy. I decided to lie to Lucas. I told him: 'Lucas the dreaded disease affects everyone. I too am HIV-positive. I only look healthy because I am on [antiretroviral] treatment.'

One week later, Lucas phoned Custom and told him that he had been tested and was now 'taking tablets'. However, Lucas was furious when he discovered that Custom had lied to him and yelled at Custom on the phone. But Lucas later sent a text message on his mobile phone, expressing a wish to continue their friendship. Custom told me, 'HIV needs positive thinking. If you do not think positively it will destroy you.'

Residents of Impalahoek still refrained from announcing at funerals that AIDS-related diseases had been the cause of death. But there were now instances in which the representatives of political and civic organisations spoke about AIDS in general terms, when they made announcements about events in the community at the graveyard. For example, a municipal councillor announced that people should not claim that others had bewitched them when they were ill but should test for HIV antibodies. He emphasised that the ANC could assist in securing fruit and vegetables for them, should they be infected with the 'dreaded disease'.

Conclusions

In this chapter, I have warned against the assumption that confessional technologies – such as coming out with an HIV-positive identity – provide a universally appropriate means of confronting the AIDS pandemic. Confessional technologies are premised on the assumption that speech has the capacity to combat stigma and bring new hope in the context of suffering and pain. These assumptions accord with classical anthropological observations that the potency of ritual lies as much in the uttering of words as in the manipulation of material objects (Malinowski 1966; Tambiah 1968). This recalls Lévi-Strauss's (1963) classical analysis of how South American shamans use songs and chants to heal cases of problematic childbirth during the *cuna* ritual. The songs relay a mystical journey that the shaman embarks upon to retrieve the woman's soul from the underworld. For Lévi-Strauss, the words of the songs are effective on a symbolic level: they resonate with the woman's chaotic struggles, name her pains, and place them in a meaningful conceptual framework, thereby making them sufferable. The words combat hopelessness by imposing order and bringing conflicts to a level of consciousness where they can be addressed (ibid.).

But, as we have seen, words can also be deadly. They also have the capacity to invoke negative emotions such as jealousy and scorn and bring about harmful effects. In insecure rural areas, such as Bushbuckridge and Venda, concealment and silence have continued to be the predominant responses to HIV and AIDS (McNeill and Niehaus 2009). Here, anxiety about the destructive capacity of words – as in cursing, swearing, and direct speech about sex and death – was overpowering. The words 'HIV' and 'AIDS' bore a negative symbolic load and prophesised death. Being pronounced 'HIV-positive' was more likely to provoke scorn and stigma than compassion.

Words operate in different social and material contexts. In West Africa and in South African urban areas, AIDS activists might well use confessional technologies as a means of forging social support, accessing medication and attaining the benefits of therapeutic citizenship (Nguyen 2010; Fassin et al. 2008). In West Africa, telling a good story and establishing a persona as a responsible patient might well have been a crucial strategy for securing access to scarce and unevenly available antiretroviral medication. In this context, the situation in places such as Bushbuckridge was very different. Prior to 2005, effective medication was out of reach of everyone suffering from AIDS-related sicknesses. After this date it was theoretically available to all. As such, confession did not necessarily confer any benefits. In this context, it was the policies of government, and their implementation, rather than the performances of potential patients that secured access to therapeutic resources.

In Impalahoek, it makes greater sense to treat speech and silence as alternative, perhaps equally appropriate, modes of dealing with disease. It is imperative that health workers learn to deal with silence, maintain confidentiality and speak with discretion.

5
Knowledge

During my visit to Impalahoek in August 2005 (the year in which ARVs were first made available through public healthcare facilities), I found Reginald (Reggie) Ngobeni to be desperately ill. The cousin of a research assistant, he had recently returned from Johannesburg and suffered from the familiar symptoms of AIDS. Reggie was extremely thin, coughed, had lesions on his body, and could hardly walk. Yet instead of testing for HIV antibodies and seeking biomedical care, he saw his symptoms as being due to spirit possession and was undergoing training as a diviner's apprentice. Although I asked Reggie's brother to take him to hospital, I was not optimistic about his chances of recovery.

I again visited the Ngobeni family in July 2007, almost two years later, and was prepared for the worst. I was therefore extremely surprised when Reggie greeted me at the gate. He appeared to be in perfect health and was busy cultivating a new patch of vegetables in his mother's yard, where he now lived. Reggie said that he had made a miraculous recovery since he joined the ZCC, and that he drank tea and coffee prescribed by the Holy Spirit. Later, he told me that he had also been taking HAART but remained adamant that it was the ZCC and not the nurses at the Rixile clinic that healed him.

Reggie felt lonely and welcomed company. He was therefore eager, during the next two weeks, to tell his cousin and me about his experiences of sickness and recovery. While listening attentively to his detailed accounts of the diviners, churches, hospitals and clinics he consulted, and about the herbs and drugs he used, it dawned on me that his narratives might bear important lessons for anthropological notions of therapeutic efficacy in contexts of medical pluralism (Janzen 1978; Olsen and Sargent 2017) and poly-ontological beliefs (Scott 2007). They lead us to reconsider simplistic correlations between 'treatment literacy' and successful adherence to antiretroviral therapy.

Following the roll-out of HAART by South African public health facilities in 2005, the focus of scholars and activists has shifted from challenging an obnoxious government to examining the knowledge and behaviour of consumers, and potential consumers, of HAART. The new focus echoes the concern with 'patient empowerment' and 'self-responsibility' in the 'new public health movement' (Lupton and Petersen 1996). It also resonates with the scholarly emphasis on rights and responsibilities of 'therapeutic citizenship' (Nguyen 2010; Robins 2006). From these perspectives, the uptake of HAART, and adherence to therapy, is a product of information, motivation and skills operating at the level of the individual (Ware et al. 2009: 45).[1] Health activists and scholars frequently deploy the concept of 'treatment literacy' to explain variations in this regard (Nachega et al. 2005). The concept denotes the capacity of infected persons not only to use ARVs effectively, but also to 'interpret information about HIV/AIDS prevention, testing and care' and 'prevent HIV/AIDS-related stigma and discrimination' (Schenker 2006: 3).

Health activists regularly conflate the effective use of ARVs with general education and with a commitment to biomedical models. The participants at an international summit on HIV/AIDS held in Cape Town during 2003 emphasised that 'education is as important as medicine' (Schenker 2006: 26). Several studies posit a robust association between health knowledge and 'therapeutic efficacy', understood as adherence to treatment and suppression of viral replication (Bangsberg et al. 2001).[2]

In this context, education for HIV/AIDS prevention, testing and care has become an emerging professional field. After having fought for the provision of ART by public healthcare facilities for more than a decade, South Africa's TAC entered a new phase of activism by vigorously implementing treatment literacy programmes. A central question has been 'how to signify concepts of the virus, immune system and anti-retroviral drugs for people with limited education and limited exposure to biomedical theories of disease' (Ashforth and Natrass 2005: 285). The TAC teaches conventional scientific understandings. At workshops throughout the country, the campaign's treatment literacy practitioners explicitly use the language of biomedicine to convey information about immunology, microbiology, treatment, CD4 counts and legal rights (ibid.: 297). They reject information arising from alternative remedies and understandings of HIV and AIDS and make a concerted attempt to democratise science. Knowledge is presented as a means of empowerment, and participants are encouraged to document how social worlds, interpersonal violence and HIV affect their bodies (MacGregor 2009). By contrast, the KwaZulu-Natal Department of Health harnesses 'indigenous knowledge' in HIV/AIDS counselling. Its culturally sensitive audiovisual material compares HIV to 'poisonous snakes' and portrays the immune system as 'body soldiers' (Ashforth and

Natrass 2005). To date, no study has assessed the efficacy of these different languages of prevention.[3]

In this chapter, I explore how the social life of ARVs intersects with the biography of Reggie Ngobeni. In doing so, I aim to contribute to ongoing debates by demonstrating that a far more complex and uneven relationship exists between 'therapeutic literacy' and 'therapeutic efficacy' than many health activists assume. First, I contend that in the village setting a plethora of social and material factors that have little to do with knowledge affect the uptake of and successful adherence to HAART. The political failure to authorise ARVs, inadequate infrastructure, stigma, alternative sickness aetiologies, extreme poverty and everyday constructs of masculinity might all inhibit the effective provision of adequate medication. Given these barriers, treatment literacy might not necessarily imply therapeutic efficacy. Second, I seek to demonstrate how, in contexts of radical medical pluralism, the lives of individuals with HIV, such as Reggie Ngobeni, are characterised by multiple, continuously shifting understandings of sickness and healing, which make 'treatment literacy' extremely hard to assess. Moreover, Reggie's biography shows how people can effectively use ARVs in the absence of any firm commitment to biomedical perspectives on HIV/AIDS.

Social and material barriers

Health activists engaged in the promotion of 'therapeutic literacy' frequently underestimate the extent to which people in rural areas, such as the villages of Bushbuckridge, have been exposed to biomedical perspectives on HIV and AIDS. As noted in the first three chapters of this book, in the early years of the pandemic, public health workers, NGOs such as LoveLife, and teachers made concerted efforts in the fields of AIDS awareness and education.

The availability of HAART has not displaced the earlier emphasis on pedagogy. The Rixile HIV clinic offered very comprehensive treatment literacy programmes. All persons who tested for HIV antibodies received extensive pre- and post-test counselling. Nurses asked everyone who tested 'HIV-positive' to choose a definite time of day for taking ARVs, and then provided clear instructions on their use. They also underlined the importance of adherence, informed patients about the actual and potential side effects of ARVs, and advised them on how to disclose their status to others. Each month, when patients at the clinic collect their medication, they have to attend compulsory HIV support group meetings. Mfecane (2010: 201) observes that facilitators at the clinic did not enable open dialogue, but instead sought to implant 'new biological discourse' into attendants. They instructed all patients to eat healthily and never to use 'traditional medicines'. The facilitators also lambasted popular pursuits such as smoking, drinking and multiple sexual liaisons. Attendants explicitly referred to the meetings as 'lessons' and to the facilitators as 'teachers'.

Not only do healthcare activists underestimate the currency of biomedical aetiologies about HIV and AIDS in local knowledge, their emphasis on 'treatment literacy' also distracts attention from features of the broader social, political and economic environments that impact upon the uptake of HAART. Foremost among these factors is the failure of President Thabo Mbeki's government to authorise ARVs (Biehl 2007) and to establish an effective infrastructure for their delivery. However, commentators seldom acknowledge that President Mbeki's mistaken views about the nature of HIV also drew on the biomedical sciences. During the late 1990s, for example, Mbeki's cabinet pinned its hopes on a 'miracle drug' called Virodene, developed at Pretoria Academic Hospital (Fassin 2007: 41–9). President Mbeki's later denial of the existence of HIV was also based on the views of dissident scientists, whose recommendations of improved sanitation and nutrition were well-established public health initiatives (Gevisser 2009: 315–33). His Health Minister, Manto Tshabalala-Msimang, expressed her opposition to ARVs in the language of biomedicine. For example, she claimed that AZT (azidothymidine) 'attacked inoffensive microbes', and she opposed nevirapine not simply because of its cost but also because it produced side effects, did not combine well with tuberculosis medication, and offered no protection against HIV transmission by breastfeeding (Fassin 2007: 82–5). Tshabalala-Msimang's failure to endorse HAART, even after the public sector roll-out had begun, was also based on its alleged 'toxicity'. These examples show that the adoption of elements of a scientific viewpoint per se is not any guarantee of the adoption of appropriate health policies that serve the needs of the population at large.

Other social and economic factors operating in village settings might also facilitate or inhibit effective treatment. Expectations of stigma and ostracism have discouraged sick persons from testing for HIV antibodies. Even urban TAC activists who disclose their status at public events prefer not to do so in their home communities (Ashforth and Natrass 2005: 293). As we have seen, such stigma is a product of different discourses, including the initial presentation in public health propaganda of AIDS as an incurable condition. Saying that a person was afflicted with a potentially deadly condition might generate a fatalistic attitude and raise questions about whom he or she might have infected. HAART reduced some – but not all – fears of stigma and feelings of guilt.

A second factor that might discourage the effective use of ARVs is the presence of plausible alternative interpretations of sickness. As we saw in Chapter 3, diviners and Christian healers might well interpret what physicians diagnose as symptoms of AIDS as signs of bewitchment. Ashforth (2002) argues that the association of AIDS with witchcraft is particularly appealing in contexts of social inequality, where virtually anyone is capable of envy. As we have seen, attributions of witchcraft counters victim-blaming by shifting responsibility from the afflicted person onto others, such as neighbours.

Third, extreme poverty has undermined treatment regimes. Unemployed men have significantly higher rates of non-adherance with HAART (Bhat et al. 2010: 951). People who register a CD4 count of 350 (previously 200) or lower are judged incapable of working and are entitled to receive disability grants.[4] Valued at R780 (approximately £50) per month in 2005, these grants were a significant source of income in many households. In this context, hospital patients used poor health as a bargaining chip to negotiate for income. Based on her enquiries in KwaZulu-Natal, Leclerc-Madlala (2006) claims that some patients would rather be HIV-positive with money than HIV-negative without money. Her research participants constantly feared losing their grant money once their health improved, and some defaulted on taking medication to drive down their CD4 cell counts.

Fourth, as in so many other dimensions of life in South Africa, gendered concerns come into play. Throughout the country, men are two times less likely than women to verify their HIV status (Government of South Africa 2010), and, once on treatment, they are more likely to default on treatment. During 2008, men constituted only 33 per cent of people receiving antiretroviral treatment at the Rixile clinic (MacPherson et al. 2008: 589). Men were by no means eager participants in support group meetings at the clinic; they usually sat in the rear and concealed their doubts about the proceedings (Mfecane 2011: 132). Researchers attribute this gendered disparity to men's general reluctance to adopt the 'sick' role, but also to the fact that health services are predominantly staffed by women nurses, who are more accommodating to the concerns of women patients (Skhosana et al. 2006). There is also a strong association between non-adherence to HAART and the consumption of alcohol (Dahab et al. 2011: 58), an important component of masculine sociability (Mager 2010).

The existence of these factors undermines the optimistic view that the mere teaching of biomedical perspectives would necessarily produce appropriate results. Even 'therapeutically literate' patients had to contend with the absence of support from the government they helped to elect, and on whose redistributive policies they relied. They, too, experienced social stigma and a chronic lack of money, and might be compelled to renegotiate gendered identities. These costs sometimes outweighed the benefits that adherence to courses of therapy might bring.

There are also factors operating in local settings that might encourage the effective uptake and use of ARVs. As we have seen, the medicalisation of women's bodies might well facilitate adherence to treatment regimes. Moreover, the existence of broad and diffuse kinship networks in sub-Saharan Africa might provide resources and social support that enable people to access HAART (Ware et al. 2009).

The life story of Reginald Ngobeni

I have selected the life story of Reginald Ngobeni for presentation because of the special vividness of his descriptions, rather than for the uniqueness of his experiences. Reggie's accounts of his own life experiences bring to light different social factors relevant to the uptake and use of ARVs among men of his generation. Beyond confirming the importance of having to confront the issue of culpability at the level of interpersonal relations, it highlights an indeterminacy of knowledge. In Impalahoek, the diagnosis and labelling of sickness commonly involved the consultation of diverse specialists, such as diviners, Christian healers and different biomedical practitioners, as well as constantly shifting, but nonetheless coexisting, perspectives on sickness.

Reggie, who contracted HIV while working in the lower echelons of the Johannesburg labour market, successfully used HAART in a profoundly pluralistic context. His accounts show how 'therapeutic efficacy' can be attained without any firm commitment to clinical aetiologies of HIV and AIDS, and in the absence of 'treatment literacy' as understood in conventional biomedical terms.

Coming of age in Bushbuckridge, 1961–88

Reggie Ngobeni was born in the village of Calcutta in the former Gazankulu Bantustan. He was the third son of his father's first wife, Maria Mathebula, and described his domestic unit as 'nearly wealthy'. By local standards this seems to be an accurate description of their economic status. His father's two wives each had sufficient land to cultivate maize, peanuts and sugarcane, and to let a large herd of cattle and goats graze. But the traumatic death of Reggie's father in 1966 tore the extended family apart. His remaining paternal kin accused his mother of witchcraft, and tensions became so severe that she felt compelled to relocate to Impalahoek, then located in the Lebowa Bantustan. Reggie therefore encountered mystical explanations for misfortune early in life. In retrospect, he believed that his mother was innocent, and that his paternal kin made the accusation in a bid to claim inheritance of his father's property.

Reggie and his brothers accompanied their mother. In Impalahoek, the Mathebula family formed part of a sizeable Shangaan minority. Here, Reggie resided with his mother, his grandmother, two older siblings (Petrus and Sidney), and later also with his two half-siblings (Steven and Aaron). His half-siblings were the progeny of men with whom his mother established relations in Impalahoek. Both Steven and Aaron used the surname Ngobeni rather than those of their own fathers. They did this to facilitate the equivalence and solidarity of the sibling group (Niehaus 2013: 38–9).

Reggie attended local schools, but only from 1971 until 1977. He seemed to have done fairly well but dropped out during his first year of secondary school. Reggie attributed this to poverty. His maternal kin had no rural resources, and the Mathebula men working in South Africa's urban and industrial centres as migrants seldom sent remittances to his mother and grandmother. 'It was really difficult to be without a father. Nobody worked at home. At school I had no books, no shoes and no [school] uniform.'

Neighbours alerted me to another reason why Reggie quit school. In 1976, the year of the national uprisings, several political activists had fled Soweto for Impalahoek to evade the police, and his grandmother accommodated them in a building in her backyard. Some of the political refugees were renowned football players. Others possessed firearms and engaged in crime. Reggie was constantly seen in the company of these men and, according to neighbours, assisted them in criminal operations, such as looting general dealer stores and stealing livestock, equipment and machinery from white-owned farms.

Reggie was eager to recount how the men from Soweto taught him about politics, and about heroes of the liberation struggle such as Steve Biko and Nelson Mandela. Although he did not say a word about crime, he boasted that he was a lucky gambler and once won R1,000 (£80) in a single card game. He attributed his success to the use of potions that he obtained from an elderly male relative. Reggie had sufficient money to send his younger half-siblings to school – whether that money came from the proceeds of crime or from gambling. While Steven completed high school, Aaron dedicated himself to liberation movements and to the anti-apartheid struggle. During 1990, Aaron was part of a small group of young men who crossed the Mozambican border to undergo training as soldiers of the ANC's military wing, MK (uMkhonto we Sizwe or 'Spear of the Nation'). Aaron sent two letters home from Zambia, but never returned from exile, and he has been missing ever since.

As a young man, Reggie enjoyed good health but occasionally suffered from excruciating stomach cramps. He first experienced these cramps on Christmas day, 1980. 'My stomach became sore,' he said. 'It was so painful. I fell down and rolled from the pain. I felt pain whenever I moved my body. It felt as if there was something hot, burning inside my stomach.' Reggie failed to identify the precise source of his distress. He encountered two contrasting accounts for the cause of his sickness. A diviner attributed his symptoms to possession by fierce Ndzau spirits, who called him to undergo training as a diviner-herbalist. During training, the spirit is exhorted to state its demands and, once appeased, can be converted to a benevolent force.[5] By contrast, an Apostolic healer revealed that neighbours had bewitched Reggie. She lit candles and prayed for him. Reggie appreciated these interventions and gained relief from the pain, but he did not know which diagnosis to believe. Reggie was therefore compelled to live with indeterminacy. Such confusion about the precise source of one's distress contradicts the implicit assumption in many social surveys that health-seekers display an unswerving commitment to a single interpretative paradigm (Helman 1984).

Life, love and sex in Johannesburg, 1988–96

In 1988, at the age of 27, Reggie left home to search for work in Johannesburg. He idealised Johannesburg as a place of political power and wealth, but given his poor education, Reggie could only hope to gain employment on the lower echelons of the city's labour market. At first, he secured accommodation in Meadowlands in the garage of Milton Nonyane and his father, who were also from Impalahoek.

He paid only R150 (£13) per month in rent and was happy that the garage was 'not too cold'. Reggie later found it more convenient to stay in Soweto with an old man called Mabetha Matlale, whose son had once resided in his grandmother's compound in Impalahoek. He paid no rent, but he regularly bought the old man groceries, meat and home-brewed liquor. Reggie soon found work at an engineering company that repaired mining technology. He was very happy with his wage of R250 (£20) per week after deductions but complained bitterly about the foul smell of the grease he had to remove from the machines. The smell, he said, constantly made him feel nauseous.

In Soweto, Reggie fell in love for the first time – with Zanele Maseko, a young Swazi woman. Reggie had previously engaged in sexual intercourse in Impalahoek. He said that on a few occasions women had asked him to accompany them and invited him to their rooms. But Reggie was anxious about women's company and feared that sexual intercourse might pollute his gambling potions and render them ineffective. He also told me that he preferred to choose his own partners. Reggie's relationship with Zanele fulfilled his greatest desires: she was beautiful, contributed financially to their endeavours by working at a crèche, cooked for him and cleaned his room. 'She satisfied my heart,' he exclaimed.

The security that Reggie found in Soweto ended abruptly. In 1994, Matlale threw Reggie out of his home for swearing and fighting with others in the early morning hours. He and Zanele then rented a room for R150 (£13) per month. But, in February 1995, Reggie lost his job at the engineering company. His technical director reportedly fired him because he had become obsessively interested in politics after Nelson Mandela's release from prison, and regularly attended trade union meetings: 'He [the director] said that I was a rotten potato, who made the other potatoes to be rotten.'

In the same year that Reggie became unemployed, Zanele left him for another man, called Findo. There is a definite economy of sexual relations, in which men who are unable to provide resources to their partners find themselves in an extremely vulnerable position. Reggie was deeply hurt by the experience of rejection and began to question his status as a man. Not only did he fail to provide financially for his lover, he also began to doubt whether he had been able to satisfy Zanele sexually. Reggie suspected that he might well be infertile; he desperately wanted to father a child and never used condoms during sexual intercourse but had failed to impregnate Zanele: 'Findo took my girlfriend in 1996, and he made her pregnant in 1997 ... After losing her, I hated everything.'

In July 1997, Reggie found a new position as an assistant and security guard at Cardies – a shop that sold birthday, wedding, Valentine's day and Christmas cards, as well as gifts such as glass. The shop was located in downtown Johannesburg. He worked from Monday to Saturday and earned only R150 (£13) per week. Reggie commented that this position provided him with the opportunity to meet new lovers, and told me that he engaged in numerous sexual liaisons to regain his lost masculine status:

> I used to proposition every beautiful girl who came into the shop. The girls came to choose cards. It was really not too difficult to grab them. Many of them accepted. At lunch, we would go to the flat of one of my friends in Plein Street [to have sex] and at night we would sleep at my own place. I really don't know how many women I had, but it was a lot. It happened every day. Some days I had two women: one in the day and one at night. It was more than 80 or 100. My friends said that I was the principal of girls because I changed them so often. I tried to satisfy my painful heart. I did not prevent because I was looking for a child. Most of the time I ate flesh to flesh [had unprotected sex]. I only used condoms when the girls wanted it.

Reggie worked at Cardies for only 18 months. In 1998 the shop became insolvent and closed down. He said that this was because black people do not really buy cards.

In 1998, Reggie befriended Clifford Mnisi, who was once President Mandela's bodyguard and knew a great deal about politics. A Portuguese man asked them to look after his home in southern Johannesburg, near the well-known George Gough migrant hostel, while he was abroad. But the homeowner never returned. There were rumours that he was a fugitive from the police, and also that Reggie had forged documents showing that the Portuguese man had in fact sold the home to him. Clifford assisted Reggie in finding a new position as a security guard at an Eskom (Electricity Supply Commission) PayPoint in a shopping mall. The position paid R1,500 (£125) per month but was extremely dangerous. Masked men with assault rifles twice robbed shops in the mall. Again, Reggie had opportunities to meet lovers:

> It was the same in the shopping mall as at Cardies. The girls were still there. During the day I screwed them at the RDP [Reconstruction and Development Programme] homes at George

Gough, and at night they slept at my home. I would go with one at lunch and take another one later. Then, tomorrow I would take more syrup [lovers]. All the time I did it flesh to flesh. I wanted to show that Zanele meant nothing to me. I used to screw all the nations: Shangaan, Pedi, Swazi, Venda, Ndebele, Zulu and Xhosa.

Reggie's friends who visited him in Johannesburg confirmed to me that he had had many lovers. They believed that this was because he could offer them appropriate accommodation near the George Gough hostel.

Experiencing illness and misfortune, 2001–04

In Johannesburg, Reggie periodically experienced illness, and his stomach cramps became progressively more severe. During 1996, his health problems came to a head when he developed a blistering fever. Reggie returned to Impalahoek to consult a Christian healer. She told him that his blood was polluted because he had broken a taboo – he had had sexual intercourse with a woman who had recently aborted and was therefore in a state of extreme heat (fiša). The healer cut a cross in his hair, rubbed soap on his head, and melted it with a red-hot steel poker. This technique presumably made the heat escape from his body.

However, Reggie suspected that there might well be deeper, more profound reasons for his distress. This was because his physical illness coincided with other forms of misfortune. In 2001, Reggie was again dismissed from work, and was also the victim of violence. On one occasion he and a friend became involved in a fist fight with Zulu men at a tavern. The Zulu men overpowered them and knocked out two of his friend's teeth with gold fillings. On another occasion, coloured men[6] robbed Reggie and threw him into a dam. Biomedical aetiologies of disease do not address the co-occurrence of sickness and other forms of misfortune, and Reggie again sought recourse to spiritual healing. A diviner instructed Reggie to sacrifice a goat in order to thank his ancestors for having enabled him to survive these ordeals. An Apostolic healer revealed that misfortune (bati) contaminated Reggie's body. He asked Reggie to place an old bronze coin, mutton fat and a chicken egg in a basin, to pour water on top, and to wash himself with the concoction. She then prayed for Reggie and asked him to hide the egg in tall grass, pour out the water in the form of a cross, and walk away without looking back.

Two years later, Reggie was once again struck down by excruciating stomach pains. He could not comprehend what was happening to his body. Reggie heard many rumours and conspiracy theories about HIV and AIDS (see Chapter 2).

> In Johannesburg people started talking about AIDS. They told us not to use the small street next to the Carlton Hotel. This is because there were thugs. They had syringes and would put HIV on your buttocks, so that you would later get AIDS. They also stopped us from eating navel oranges because they said the farmers put AIDS in those oranges. Later they said a sore with a black spot is a sign of AIDS. My friends said that Basson [Dr Wouter Basson, head of the apartheid government's chemical weapons programme] came here with the disease. AIDS is like Ebola. It kills people. I wanted to know from other friends where AIDS comes from. They said it was in condoms.

However, Reggie did not believe that he had been infected with HIV. He reasoned that his sickness commenced during 1980, well before the onset of the pandemic. Because he had been away from home for more than 16 years, Reggie feared that he had become alienated from his kin and ancestors. His lack of spiritual protection had rendered him vulnerable to mystical attacks, such as witchcraft, and he felt that it was essential that he should reconstruct his fractured social and spiritual relations. Reggie was now in a desperate situation. He was unemployed and extremely ill, and friends such as Clifford were no longer able or prepared to support him.

The quest for therapy in Impalahoek, 2004–06

On 27 April 2004, Reggie's younger half-brother, Aaron, came to fetch him by car and took him back to his mother's home in Impalahoek. Reggie told me that he constantly felt exceptionally tired, as if he had lifted heavy cement slabs. He initially suspected that his maternal aunt might have bewitched him. She apparently swore at him because he had not visited her for more than 15 years.

Afisi Khomane, his sister-in-law, was a diviner, and she tried to nurse him back to health. Afisi insisted that Ndzau spirits had afflicted Reggie and were calling him to become a diviner. These spirits usually strike the stomach. Afisi thus arranged for her mother, who was an instructor of diviners (*gobela*), to train him. Reggie's mother and siblings raised R3,500 (£290) for his apprenticeship, and also provided a tonne of wood, an 80-kilogram bag of maize meal, a 12-kilogram bag of sugar, a blanket and a chicken for the rituals he had to undergo. Reggie's instructor helped him frame his suffering in a meaningful conceptual and discursive framework. She told him that no fewer than five different spirits manifested themselves while he was in a trance. But Reggie's training did not ease his physical discomfort. In fact, his pains grew worse.

One morning, after Reggie had been to the toilet, his intestines protruded from his anus. His instructor was shaken and felt compelled to ask his brother, Petrus, to take him to Tintswalo hospital. There, nurses and doctors diagnosed him as suffering from tuberculosis. He felt extremely disconcerted that they disregarded his own accounts of his symptoms and based their diagnosis purely on the statements of his instructor and the results of diagnostic tests. Although nearly half of all tuberculosis patients at Tintswalo hospital were co-infected with HIV (Pronyk 2001: 620), Reggie claimed that medical personnel did not test him for HIV antibodies. This is hard to believe, and it seems more likely that medical personnel offered to test him and that he declined.

Reggie was confined to the tuberculosis ward for just over three weeks. He described the ward as a polluted space of death, with little water and food, and bleak prospects of recovery:

Each morning they [the hospital nurses] woke us at six o'clock and gave me two tablets. Then we had to wash ourselves. But there was no water in the taps in our ward, and the nurses would bring water in buckets. You had to buy your own soap, washing rag, and Vaseline. I did not wash because the space for washing was too small and because I don't like standing naked with others. In the TB ward, I wore cloth for the spirits. The nurses told me to take it off, but I refused. My mattress stank. It had the bad smell of urine.

At teatime, they usually gave us tea and bread. Sometimes it was different. Then we would get Jungle Oats [porridge]. This is number one. Visiting time was from ten o'clock to half past ten [in the morning], and again from two o'clock till three [during the afternoon]. There was nothing in the evening. If you wanted to eat, you had to bring your own food. Each day there was a preacher, who preached and told us the word of God.

More than six people died in the ward when I was there. One of them died this side of my bed. The next one died that side of my bed. They [the clinical staff] brought other patients, but they also died. They put something like a tent at the place where someone had died and removed the dead body with a noisy trolley. I was so scared. I feared that I might follow them. I shivered. After the deaths, there is a bad aura [seriti] and I feared that the aura might come to me. I was afraid. In that ward, you never knew who would die next.

While in hospital, Reggie dreamed of a large snake with seven heads. It flew in a strong wind and settled in the trees above his head. The snake instructed him not to take his medication and promised to show him money. Reggie was not sure what to make of the dream. In Impalahoek, people viewed snakes as anomalous creatures. As animals from below the ground, where the deceased are buried, they were messengers from the ancestors and could also be omens of death. In addition, residents associated snakes with water and with precious metals, which were sources of wealth, but also causes of conflict and murder. Such revelatory dreams, as we shall see, are highly significant repositories of meaning in the context of sickness.

After being discharged from hospital, Reggie resumed his training as a diviner. He anxiously defied the snake of his dreams and continued taking his tuberculosis medication. Although he still felt weak, he was compelled to display great endurance. Reggie had to wake up early each morning, invoke the spirits to greet visitors, and dig roots and herbs in the forest. He complained that his legs felt dry, and that he could no longer dance properly. Grave tensions soon emerged between Reggie and his instructor. He blamed her for making contradictory statements. All along she had said that spirits affected Reggie's legs. But now she proclaimed that he had trampled on a potion (called *sefolane*) that witches laid in the path he used when walking to the shop to purchase cold drinks. His instructor constantly demanded more money and reportedly warned Reggie that he could be struck down with AIDS if he did not pay her. This statement amounted to a curse: 'I cried when I heard those painful words.'

Reggie, nonetheless, endured the pain, danced, and graduated as a diviner on 31 May 2005. By now, he said, his family had paid his instructor nearly R15,000 (£1,250) for her services.

Using ARVs in Impalahoek, 2005–10

Back at his mother's home from the diviner's compound, Reggie again became terribly ill:

As I entered the yard of my mother's home everything turned upside down. I started to be sick again. I slept in a tent outside, vomited, and coughed throughout the night. It was so painful in my chest. I also had diarrhoea and my nose bled. I thought that I was dying.

During this time his instructor's apprentices (*matwasane*) came to dance for him, and relatives rubbed ointment on his legs. In June 2005, Reggie consulted a general practitioner, who, he said, did not test him for HIV antibodies, but merely prescribed tablets and told him to eat boiled, rather than fried, eggs.

Eventually Petrus took his ailing brother to the Rixile clinic. Reggie told me that it was not his decision to consult the nurses at the clinic. 'I had heard of Rixile and did not want to go there, but Petrus wanted to know what was bugging me.' This compromise shows that decisions on therapeutic consultations are seldom those of individual sick persons themselves, as social surveys often presume. Instead, such decisions are the outcome of complex negotiations within therapy management groups – networks of carers, kin and affines – who mobilise around the sufferer to support them, decide on treatments, and collectively evaluate the outcome of therapy (see Janzen 1978).

Fortunately, Reggie's encounters with the clinic provided a stark contrast to his earlier experiences in the dreaded tuberculosis ward. The clinic was within walking distance from his home and had begun to supply free HAART. In addition, the clinic provided outpatient nursing and comprehensive treatment literacy programmes and regularly monitored CD4 counts. By 2007, Rixile was catering for approximately 6,000 patients (MacPherson et al. 2008: 590). Reggie tested HIV-positive and was part of the first generation of men in Impalahoek to be placed on a regime of HAART.

Reggie's detailed descriptions of procedures at the clinic show that he rapidly acquired accurate biomedical knowledge about HIV/AIDS. When he arrived at Rixile, he said, nurses took blood from his finger, told him that he had tested HIV-positive, and measured a CD4 count of only 94, which was sufficiently low to merit anti-retroviral treatment. The nurses asked him to choose a time of day and henceforth take ARVs at 12-hour intervals. They underlined the importance of therapeutic adherence and instructed him always to use condoms during sexual intercourse, and always to use gloves when helping bleeding persons. The nurses did not raise any false hopes. Reggie explicitly told me: 'The tablets won't cure AIDS. They will only make the AIDS weaker.'

Reggie's perceptions were far more complex, contradictory and ambivalent than social surveys on treatment literacy assume to exist among health-seekers (Nachega et al. 2005). Despite being well informed on biomedical perspectives on HIV, AIDS, HAART and his own test results, Reggie could not bring himself to accept that he was really HIV-positive. He continued to suspect that his divination instructor had cursed him and had disguised the symptoms of his witchcraft-related sicknesses as AIDS.

> I don't know if they [medical personnel at the clinic] are correct. This is because I do not know what AIDS pains are like. I did not believe the doctor. I thought that my instructor had bewitched me. This is because I started vomiting and bleeding through the nose at her home. She and her child put potions and stones in the corners of my room and told me not to sweep. I did not give them permission to do so ... When someone promises you that you will get AIDS, you will remember it. I thought my instructor was responsible. I thought she gave me AIDS.

For Reggie, the acceptance of an HIV-positive diagnosis would imply culpability, not merely for bringing about his own sickness, but potentially also for having infected numerous sexual partners.

> I don't think I have HIV. I do not believe it comes from unprotected sex. I'm not HIV-positive. The disease that I have is the very same stomach cramps that started in 1980. I do not know the name of this sickness. My disease does not come from sex. By 1980 I did not have a girlfriend. My girlfriends started in 1990. If it had been AIDS, it would have killed me long ago. People with AIDS die in 15 years, not in 28 years. It is not sex. I never took dirty girls. I would only take good-looking and clean ones. Ones who wash and wear clean clothes. AIDS might be there, but I selected my girlfriends.

Nevertheless, Reggie took the ARV tablets as instructed. His reasoning expresses a fear of the power of words. In a similar manner as his instructor had cursed him, he said, the nurses at Rixile told him that unless he took ARVs he would die. Reggie feared that these words might well bring about a tragic end to his life. 'I decided to drink the tablets,' he said, 'because I'm afraid to die ... If I do not take these tablets people will lie. They will say that AIDS killed me because I did not take the tablets or follow the instructions.'

Paradoxically he interpreted the vivid and frightening dreams that are a well-known biochemical side effect of the drug efavirenz as a sign of the mysterious therapeutic power of antiretroviral medication.

The tablets made me sweat and made me dream about
dangerous things and about good things. Once I dreamed that
I was dead. I dreamed that there was a sign on the fence of my
yard saying 'REGGIE IS DEAD! PLEASE, DONATE MONEY
FOR HIS FUNERAL.' Other times I also dreamed about money.
I once dreamed that I had R266 million [£19 million]. I dreamed
that the whole plaza [shopping centre] and the substation [for
electricity] was mine. I dreamed that the ancestors had given
me these things. But it was not the ancestors – it was the tablets.
The tablets reminded me about dead people and about forgotten
things. Maybe there are drugs inside those tablets.

One dream occurred on the borderlines of sleep and wakeful-
ness, and seemed so real that it prompted Reggie to wander from his
mother's home towards a dam, approximately two kilometres away.

Once I woke up at three o'clock in the morning and I heard
voices. They called me to come to the dam. They asked me to
bring my shit to them in a bucket and they promised to give me
lots of money. I walked to the dam, but I did not find the place
[from where the voices came]. I was full of mud and I was very
tired. I heard music coming from the door of a house, and I
wanted to listen to the music. Then I entered the yard, carrying a
five-litre bucket of shit. There was a woman with a young boy and
she gave me soft porridge. She begged me to eat. She asked me
what the shit meant, and I told her that I came with the shit so
that people could give me money. She thought that witches were
trying to turn me into a zombie. I thought I was mad.

These dreams articulated Reggie's fear of death. Many diviners
see dreams of money as an omen of death. Symbolically, money is
associated with precious metals from beneath the ground, which is
also the domain of the deceased, and also with collections taken at
funerals. The desire for money might well resonate with the subcon-
scious wish for a final release from pain and suffering. Reggie,
however, observed that his health continuously improved, and that
he consistently regained weight and strength.

On 26 December 2006, Reggie received a vision from his ancestors telling him to go to the ZCC, to which his mother belonged.
Here a prophet gave him blessed water to drink and to pour at the
gate to protect his mother's home against witchcraft. The prophet
instructed Reggie to drink Joko tea, FG coffee and salt:

The prophet said that witches will send snakes to my home and that I have to kill all the snakes. So far, I have killed about 13 snakes in our yard. I found one in the shack and one underneath the drum of water in the kitchen. There was one on the kitchen door and another in between the bricks ... These are not snakes from the ancestors [*noga ya badimo*] who bring luck to the family. They are snakes from the bush who bring bad luck. They have the devil in them.

After that, Reggie attended church each Sunday and drank Zionist coffee and tea each day. This, he said, facilitated his recovery. Reggie commented on his renewed life:

When I was sick my mother did everything for me. At first, I could not wash my own clothes. I was too weak. I could not jump, and I could not walk to the plaza [shopping centre], or to church. I moved very slowly. I only became better after I went to church and took their prescriptions. Now I can walk, and I can run. I can also carry three 25-litre barrels of water, and I can plough maize in the garden. They [the ZCC] fixed [healed] my leg and the pain is better.

Reggie's most grave concern was that he had not yet received a disability pension. Nurses at the HIV clinic asked him to consult social workers and obtain an affidavit from the police station before forwarding his application. He desperately needed a regular income to purchase the proteins and vegetables that the nurses at Rixile recommended he should eat.[7]

Before parting company, we discussed the upcoming election for ANC president, to be held in Polokwane in 2009. Reggie described himself as a loyal supporter of Thabo Mbeki, then in power, whom he hoped would defeat his opponent, Jacob Zuma. His preference was not influenced by their respective policies on HIV/AIDS, but rather by ethnic stereotypes formed during his sojourn in Johannesburg. Reggie said that he did not wish to see any Zulu person elected as president, because Zulus have a reputation for tribal chauvinism and for violence. His experiences of sickness and healing stood apart from discussions in the political domain.

Reggie's life story shows how a constellation of social and economic factors that might have little to do with 'treatment literacy' affect the uptake and use of HAART. In contrast to the assumptions made by medical discourses on 'patient responsibility', his therapeutic consultations were not a product of individual knowledge. In Reggie's case they were made in consultation with his siblings, mother, sister-in-law and a divination instructor. President Mbeki's opposition to HAART constituted the backdrop to many of his experiences, but the impact of other factors was more clearly apparent. For Reggie, there were complex intellectual and emotional advantages to being a victim of pollution, witchcraft or spirit possession rather than being infected with HIV. These labels explained the early onset of his sickness and accounted for the co-occurrence of physical distress and other forms of misfortune, such as job losses. Apart from being more tolerable to oneself, these sicknesses were deemed more amenable to being cured by healers who did not operate in under-resourced rural hospitals. Financial concerns weighed more heavily in the treatment of spirit possession than witchcraft.

Reggie's life story also shows that, in situations of medical pluralism, knowledge about sickness does not imply unswerving commitment to one set of beliefs. He constantly tried out and added new concepts, and practical considerations often outweighed explanatory consistency. Different specialised authorities – diviners, Christian healers, politicians, general practitioners and HIV clinicians – acted as guarantors for the status of facts. In such contexts, healing is understood in terms of constantly changing meanings and expectations (Etkin 1991). Biomedicine itself comprises different coexisting and competing paradigms (Helman 1984). Reggie consulted a general practitioner and was treated for tuberculosis without being tested for HIV antibodies. The acceptance of alternative accounts of his illness did not prevent him from carefully adhering to prescriptions regarding the use of ARVs. His dream experiences attested to their power. The therapeutic milieu that Reggie found in the ZCC complemented HAART by providing social support, faith, and a powerful religious rationale for health maintenance.

Conclusions

The evidence presented in this chapter sounds a cautionary note in relation to existing interventions in the field of public health that emphasise the responsibility of individual patients (Lupton and Petersen 1996). As I have shown, there might well be clear limitations to strategies aimed at investing scarce resources in treatment literacy, and in promoting the uptake and successful use of HAART.

Such thinking inappropriately treats medical meanings outside the contexts of social and bodily experiences,[8] and detracts attention from the broader backdrop to AIDS, and from political, economic and social barriers to therapy. Moreover, an approach centred on the teaching of biomedical knowledge often makes untested assumptions that target populations are ignorant about biomedical models of HIV/AIDS; that there is a clear consensus within biomedicine; and that other therapeutic practices are incompatible with the effective use of HAART. These assumptions are frequently mistaken and might well impede the effective delivery of healthcare.

Authoritative instructions are clearly necessary for the effective use of ARVs (Ware et al. 2009). However, comparative studies show a contradictory, sometimes unexpected, statistical relationship between educational status, HIV infection and the outcomes of HAART. In sub-Saharan Africa, education has not inhibited the spread of HIV. Some countries with relatively high literacy rates also have high HIV prevalence rates. In 2006, literacy in South Africa was 86.4 per cent and HIV prevalence 21.5 per cent. The comparative figures in neighbouring Mozambique were 47.8 per cent and 12.2 per cent (Schenker 2006: 17). Whereas a study of one well-resourced workplace HAART programme shows a definite association between fewer years in education and poorer treatment outcomes (Dahab et al. 2011), another study of a community-based programme shows that treatment failure was most common among people with tertiary education (Bhat et al. 2010: 947). These findings suggest that health knowledge and educational attainment are not necessarily the most important determinants of HIV prevention and treatment efficacy. Complex social and cultural factors pertaining to the local settings of these programmes seem to contribute to the production of these discrepant outcomes. The biography of Reggie Ngobeni is significant insofar as it suggests what some of these factors might be.

6
Dreams

Jane Nyalungu, an instructor of diviners, tested positive for HIV antibodies during 2004, when she was in her mid-thirties. But she only sought therapy at the Rixile clinic eight years later. By then, Jane had become severely ill: she felt exceptionally weak and slept nearly all day long, and the gums of her teeth were swollen and bled profusely. Her boyfriend, who was a teacher, denied that he had infected her with HIV and terminated their relationship. In 2012, clinic staff informed Jane that her CD4 count was only 124, and immediately placed her on a regimen of HAART. They told her about all the possible side effects of the medication. Jane's sister, who was a home-based carer, came to stay with Jane to provide her with social and moral support.

Nonetheless, Jane failed to anticipate how the drugs would affect her body and mind. 'I think the tablets burst – it was as if they were bombing my body. They made me drunk and I saw many different things.'

'The first night,' she recalled, 'I heard a sound – like someone breaking furniture in my home.' The next morning Jane went to investigate, but to her surprise found that nothing had been broken. Subsequently, she experienced the following sequence of perplexing dreams.

> I dreamed that my friend Thandi got married and I passed by her wedding. I saw many children playing. There were hundreds of them. I asked 'Can't you see it's my friend's wedding?' and chased them [away]. I chased them all night long, but they kept returning and laughing at me. [In real life, Thandi is single and has only one child.]

A few nights later, Jane saw a body of poisonous green water in her dream.

> Two men came towards me. Each held me by an arm and pushed my whole body into the water. They soaked me for some minutes. I could taste the water. It was bitter. The men then pulled me out of the water and pushed an iron [rod] from my mouth through

my anus. Next, they put me in an oven and roasted me on flames. I turned, like a chicken [being spit-roasted]. I screamed, but there was nobody to help me.

In her final dream, Jane encountered her deceased father.

He sat on the floor with his legs crossed. He held a blue plastic bag containing old, blue R100 notes, and gave me some of the money. I was excited to see my father. I wanted to call my brother and tell him that my father had returned. But then my father's looks changed, and he became angry. I saw white doves – or pigeons – on his shoulders. They came towards me and bit my face. Hereafter I could no longer see my father. It was seven o'clock in the morning. I found myself on my knees crying strange cries, and shouting, 'Father! Where are you?' I phoned my sister to tell her our father had been here, but she said it was only a hallucination.

After three weeks, Jane's nightmares ceased abruptly. She then gradually regained her energy. Her gums no longer bled, and she again woke early each morning to proceed with her daily tasks. Jane believed that the tablets not only cured her, but also bestowed upon her the ability to foresee the future through her dreams. She told my research assistant and me that she had dreamed about our visit the previous evening. In her dreams, she said, snakes were an omen of trouble, and dreams of men building homes with stone bricks foretold death.

Jane's story was by no means exceptional. It captures themes that were common to the narratives of the 19 people my research assistants and I interviewed about their experiences of using ARVs between 2008 and 2014. Previous anthropological studies, such as those by Robins (2006) and by Fassin and colleagues (2008), document how residents of Cape Town and Johannesburg portrayed HAART as a journey from near death to renewed life, and from isolation to acceptance. Many of our research participants told us that they had gained similar advantages from therapy. But they not only deployed biomedical vocabularies, associated with 'therapeutic citizenship', to describe their own experiences. In addition to speaking about physical recovery and social reintegration, they recounted bizarre and frightening, yet uniquely realistic, dream experiences. From the perspective of biomedicine, vivid dreams and nightmares are nothing more than a biochemical side effect of the compound efavirenz, which affects the central nervous system. These effects are self-limiting: they usually occur within the first few days or weeks of therapy and then resolve (Carr and Cooper 2000). From the perspective of our research participants, however, these dreams were integral to the working of all antiretroviral drugs and attested to their mystical therapeutic power.

The information that I present in this chapter seeks to build on and establish connections between two very different bodies of anthropological literature, namely those on pharmaceuticals and on dreams.

Following Appadurai's (1986) approach to the social life of things, anthropologists have explored how people give value to pharmaceuticals and how pharmaceuticals, in turn, give value to social relations. Van der Geest, Reynolds Whyte and Hardon (1996) and Van der Geest and Hardon (2003) show how pharmaceuticals circulate through distinct phases – production, marketing, distribution, purchasing, prescription and consumption – in each phase entering different networks of social relations and distinct regimes of values.[1] This paradigm allows us to discern how the meanings that consumers bestow on pharmaceuticals might well differ from those that the producers intended. Consumers classify drugs in terms of vernacular understandings of colours, or categories of 'heat' and 'coolness' (Senah 1994). Pharmaceuticals are also vehicles for identity. In China, for example, Viagra evokes an ethic of sexuality centred on individual desire (Zhang 2007). Consumers' assessments of the therapeutic efficacy of pharmaceuticals also transcend their biochemical effects. The mere act of prescription renders sickness into something concrete and communicates a concern that might well enhance patient well-being (Moerman 2002).

Beliefs in the mystical efficacy of ARVs appear to be congruent with perceptions of the spiritual underpinning of herbal medicines (Feierman 1990; Langwick 2011). Throughout South Africa, certain medicinal plants are believed to have the capacity to facilitate powerful dreams (Berglund 1976: 114),[2] and to induce visions that reveal the identity of witches (Thornton 2017: 257). A plant called *inthelezi* is taken to ensure ancestral protection (Dold and Cocks 2000). Herbs and pharmaceuticals alike are believed to work in conjunction with the words of healers, and with agencies such as the ancestors and the Holy Spirit.

In sub-Saharan Africa, as elsewhere, dreams are acknowledged to provide a self-scape (Hollan 2003; Mageo 2006) and to indicate unresolved conflicts in the dreamer (Lee 1958). However, despite the intensely personal nature of dreams, dreamers use socially shared frameworks for interpreting them. Holy (1992) described how, for the Berti of Darfur in Sudan, dream symbols indicate what the dreamer might receive: for example, a dream of a goat indicates prosperity. Berti also use the same symbols in waking life. Since Tylor's (1958 [1871]) controversial theory of animism, which states that dream experiences originally gave rise to the ideas of the soul and afterlife, anthropologists have recognised the religious significance of dreams. Jedrej and Shaw (1992) document a widespread belief that the ancestors and Holy Spirit communicate messages through dreams. Curley (1983), in turn, focuses on the narration of dreams as personal performances. He demonstrates how, for Pentecostal Christians in the Cameroon, dreams about conversion and spiritual power attest to the believer's faith and provide a 'striking repository of images' that help establish religious truth.

Below, I discuss how research participants narrated their experiences of ARV-induced dreams. I suggest that this concern arises from a general attentiveness to the content of dreams in everyday life. Residents of Impalahoek imbued certain dreams with power. They believed that dreams could potentially alert people to mystical dangers such as witchcraft, communicate the wishes of the ancestors, or contain symbols that might predict future events. In the next sections, I turn to the meanings and sequences of ARV-induced dreams. I suggest that, by speaking about the content of, and figures in, selective dreams, research participants were able to articulate private feelings, such as their fears of death, that they did not ordinarily admit to others, or even to themselves. I suggest that dream narratives generally depicted a journey, marked by dissociation from the everyday, confronting situations of danger, and being comforted by benevolent spiritual helpers. For research participants, the journey did not merely lead to physical recovery, but was also a means of mystical empowerment.

Experiencing AIDS, using HAART

The 19 people we interviewed about their experiences of sickness and therapy were all recipients of HAART at the Rixile clinic at Tintswalo hospital. Given that all research participants were well acquainted with my research assistants, they were less inhibited about speaking to us about personal issues than might otherwise have been the case. Eight research participants were men and 11 women. Their ages varied from 28 to 53 years. At the onset of sickness nearly all had been employed in the lower echelons of the labour market. The men worked as security guards, general labourers or taxi drivers; the women worked as seasonal labourers on commercial farms, sold dough cakes, operated a small telephone business, or were unemployed. Only six research participants were married and lived with their spouses. Twelve resided in domestic units that also included parents, aunts, siblings, and, in one case, only children.

At the start of sickness, interviewees encountered diffuse symptoms – aches and fevers, tinnitus, a sore throat, sudden loss of appetite, diarrhoea, numb limbs, coughing, weakness and exhaustion. These symptoms became increasingly severe and were followed by opportunistic infections such as herpes and shingles. Some perceived their bodies to be rotting away while they were still alive (McNeill and Niehaus 2009: 34).

Like Reggie Ngobeni, whose experiences I discussed in Chapter 5, ten research participants first consulted diviners or Christian healers, because they suspected mystical causes of their sickness. One participant, George Dibakwane, recalled that his paternal aunt instructed him to look for herbs. 'Tablets cannot cure you,' she said. 'You need SeSotho potions [dihlare].' Julia Monareng was convinced that a senior farmworker had bewitched her because she had rejected his sexual advances. Khotsi Nxumalo's parents suspected that he might have broken a taboo by engaging in sexual intercourse during the mourning period following his wife's death. The diviners whom they consulted administered emetics and strengthened them with steaming, while the Christian healers recommended prescriptions from the Holy Spirit. Two research participants underwent apprenticeships to become diviners. As in the case of Reggie Ngobeni, these therapies proved prohibitively expensive and ineffective.

Being pronounced 'HIV-positive' crystallised sickness and brought about fears of death. Twelve research participants were found to be co-infected with tuberculosis, and were first treated at Tintswalo hospital.[3] In the tuberculosis ward, nurses were constantly present, and patients were asked to 'drink' up to seven tablets each day.[4] They were fed regularly – soft porridge and tea in the morning; fruit and juice at noon; and a meal comprising porridge, meat or fish and vegetables in the afternoon. But conditions were bleak and research participants were traumatised by the deaths of fellow patients. (See Reggie Ngobeni's description of conditions in the tuberculosis wards in 2006 in Chapter 5.)

Medical staff at Rixile clinic always prescribed a combination of three different ARVs – known by the names stavudine, lamivudine, tenofovir DF, efavirenz and/or Stocrin. Doctors and nurses provided

fairly elaborate instructions: the drugs had to be taken at 12- or
24-hour intervals, and patients should never delay or skip medication.[5] They also warned patients about the possible side effects of
ARVs, but reassured them that these would disappear after about
three weeks.[6] Nurses advised patients to disclose their status to a
friend, spouse or relative at home, who could assist them in adhering
to treatment. After the initial meeting, patients visited Rixile clinic
each month to undergo medical check-ups, attend HIV support
group meetings and receive refills. Initially, patients sometimes
queued for medication from 6 a.m. until 2 p.m., but as the clinic
became more capable of handling a faster roll-out of medication,
waiting times drastically deceased.

The optimistic results of MacPherson et al.'s (2008) study of
treatment outcomes at Rixile clinic found that side effects did not
have an excessively negative impact on adherence to HAART.[7]
Research participants mentioned dizziness, nausea, insomnia, hallu-
cinations and swellings of the limbs as possible side effects, and saw
vivid dreams as integral to the workings of ARVs. 'Everyone taking
ARVs must have these dreams,' I was told. 'Your immune system
is down, and the tablets fight the virus. The dreams are a sign that
they are working.' These effects were anticipated. Doreen Maluleke
recalled that nurses at Rixile told her that ARVs might cause her 'to
see ghosts'. Another research participant, Dan Khosa, said: 'When
you take these tablets and go to sleep, you have been forewarned.'

The significance of everyday dreams

The focus on ARV-induced dreams was a product of general
attentiveness to dreams (*ditoro*) in everyday life. This attentiveness
preceded the advent of HIV/AIDS and was intimately linked to
the prominence of dream narration in ordinary village settings. At
an elementary level, research participants distinguished between
'mundane' and 'serious' dreams, neither of which were ARV-induced.
Mundane dreams were not of much interest and were recognised as
part of ordinary mental processes. 'Everybody dreams,' I was told.
'If you dream, your brain works. If you don't, you're dead.' These
dreams either recalled past experiences or expressed disguised
wishes. Because their meanings were self-evident, one could narrate
them to virtually anyone. One of my research assistants, a retired
teacher, often told me that he dreamed he was back at school. Likewise, a childless woman relayed that she regularly dreamed about

caring for children. She saw the dream as a means of 'wish fulfil-ment', recalling Freud's (1994 [1900]) classical theory of dreams.

Serious dreams, by contrast, were bizarre or frightening. Villagers were mindful of the possibility that their content might reveal disguised dangers, predict the occurrence of future events, or relay messages from the ancestors or the Holy Spirit. Villagers did not share such dream experiences with everyone, and particularly not with rivals or those who might potentially set out to harm them. They generally took care to narrate serious dreams only to trusted kin and friends, or to fellow church members. Because their meaning was believed to be in code, their accurate interpretation was the prov-enance of diviners or of Christian ministers. There is some affinity between divination and dream interpretation. The images of such dreams, too, generated a temporary shift to a contrary, non-normal mode of cognition (Peek 1991). Dream images were ambiguous and cryptic, they provoked debate, and they provided a transference of information. In this process, people were compelled to scrutinise known facts in the light of a new perspective (ibid.: 202).

In serious dreams, images of snakes, apes, strange lights, small people and unknown white persons might be a warning that witchcraft was at work (Niehaus et al. 2001: 129). Lebo Mnisi, a 52-year-old woman, was extremely disturbed when she dreamed that a small man chased her. 'Because you've seen me,' he shouted at her, 'you'll die!' Lebo pushed the small man into a room in which many men were seated but failed to lock the door from the outside. He thus escaped and continued to pursue her. Lebo told her daughter and consulted a diviner about her dream. The diviner confirmed Lebo's expectation that the man was a nocturnal servant, or zombie (setlotl-wane), sent by witches to harm her. The divination lots indicated that an extramarital lover of Lebo's husband might be responsible, and the diviner used herbs to fortify Lebo against witchcraft.

There were also commonly recognised figures whose appearance in dreams predicted future events. Research participants suggested that crossing rivers, picking fruit, climbing without falling, R10 notes (the green colour denotes fecundity and growth) and trees (which indicate the presence of one's ancestors) symbolised good fortune. Dreams of flight showed that nobody could harm you. But there were also many standard dream figures that predicted misfortune. A snake, I was told, foretold an encounter with enemies; eating meat, poisoning; a fire, unfavourable talk; driving cattle home, divorce (the return of bridewealth); a whirlwind, impending trouble; riding a bicycle, suffering; a flooding river, insurmountable problems; torn clothing, poverty; chameleons, sickness (the reptile staggers); and falling, defeat. Possible omens of death included coins and R20 notes (as collected at funerals), rats (because they burrow like grave diggers), nakedness (death leaves one destitute), termites (which are associated with tombs), a feast (a funeral meal), flowers (wreaths) and a pit (because it resembles a grave). Fire foretold the death of an adult (widows burn their mourning attire after the mourning period), and, for members of the Khosa family, thunder predicted the death of a maternal grandparent.

Many dreamers claimed to have received premonitions through dreams. Milton Machate, a 50-year-old man, recalled that when he was a youngster, he dreamed of a whirlwind swirling around him. But a Zionist minister had told him not to worry because, in his dream, the whirlwind left his body. A week later Milton's former girlfriend, whom he no longer loved, informed him that she was pregnant. Fortunately, from his point of view, another young man accepted paternity and agreed to marry her. What made matters complex was that the meanings of dream symbols were often unclear, and one's own dream experiences might foretell what might happen to others, and vice versa. Kaizer Manzini told me that, while he was at boarding school, he dreamed that a furious man with two vicious dogs used a tomahawk to chop him to death. The next morning, he received the sad news that his mother had died.

Villagers widely believed that spiritual agencies might manifest themselves, and/or communicate their wishers, through dreams. George Shokane, once a head teacher, recalled that he purchased a Mazda 323 sedan in 1993. That very evening he dreamed that his long-deceased father approached him in a Mercedes-Benz. 'It had an open rooftop and he wanted to give me a lift.' This dream showed his father's approval of George's purchase. In other cases, visitations by the deceased in dreams prompted descendants to erect tomb-stones at their graves.

Dreams of sickness, travelling to distant lands or therapeutic consultations might foretell that the ancestors or foreign spirits were calling one to undergo an apprenticeship as a diviner. Christians interpreted biblical images in their dreams as a calling to assume a position of religious leadership. Before Elphas Bila established the Bright Church of the Morning Star, he dreamed that he followed a star and met a rider on a white horse, as described in the book of Revelations. Elphas also saw a fire spreading towards his house, but the flames departed immediately after he prayed. The final image was of a double-edged sword descending from heaven and landing in his hands. Elphas regularly narrated these dreams during church services.

The ability to derive transcendent meaning from dreams was a valued index of spiritual power. One afternoon during the late 1990s, my research assistants introduced me to Nelius Chiloane, a part-time minister in the ZCC, whom they said was a renowned interpreter of dreams. Nelius described this ability as a blessing and told us that many years ago he had foreseen the advent of South Africa's democracy. In a dream, Nelius saw black and white children – both girls and boys – seated on long rows of benches. They faced east. Suddenly, he said, a Spitfire appeared from the north. But the plane changed into a horse with two riders – a black man seated in front, and a white man in the rear, both holding the horse's reins. The horse then disappeared into a cloud. Nelius remarked: 'At the time I did not know what the dream meant. It is only now, with the political changes happening in our country, that I realise what my dream was about.' The children, he argued, represented the future, the metamorphosis of the plane into a horse the changing of governments, and the black and white riders showed that we would all have a say in government. 'The cloud means we'll all be in one house.'

The content of ARV-induced dreams

There are both similarities and differences between ordinary serious dreams and ARV-induced dreams. Research participants regularly drew upon the same symbolic codes to interpret their meanings. But they recognised that, even though the ancestors or the Holy Spirit might also be able to communicate through ARV-induced dreams, the source of these dreams lay in pharmaceuticals. Moreover, the themes of ARV-induced dreams were often novel, and they possessed a far greater vividness than ordinary serious dreams. ARV-induced dreams were always narrated in the first person and engaged the dreamer much more directly in an existential sense. Hence, research participants saw ARV-induced dreams as serious dreams of a special kind.

Mageo's (2006; 2011) method of 'figurative analysis' provides a useful way of approaching the content of the ARV-induced dreams that we recorded. To allow analytical categories to emerge from ethnographic data, she recommends that the analyst seeks to identify central figures, images and themes manifest in a corpus of dreams. The analyst should then interrogate these, drawing on both the dreamers' own interpretations and also on larger studies of the dreamers' culture. The most regularly recurring dream themes or figures in the corpus of ARV-induced dreams that we collected were: being called by mysterious voices (five instances); seeing 'small people' (two); attending weddings (three); confronting dangerous situations (ten); encountering aggressive animals (ten); visiting graveyards and/ or attending funerals (eight); being suspended at height or wandering in another world (eight); and meeting deceased relatives (13).

We can view these figures and themes as 'public symbols' through which people articulated well-established personal feelings, fears and wishes concerning their sickness. By narrating the content of ARV-induced dreams, research participants could broach anxiety-producing topics, such as social isolation, vulnerability and death, that they might not ordinarily admit to others, or even to themselves. In this context, narrating dreams constituted a form of veiled, indirect speech that resonated with the way in which residents of Impalahoek deployed euphemisms and non-verbal language to refer to sex, death and HIV/AIDS (see Chapter 5). Research participants recounted the content of such dreams to close kin, trusted acquaintances and home-based health carers in the domestic setting, and to other patients and instructors at the meetings of support groups. Their intention was not to warn others about what might happen in the future or to bid for social status, as in the case of ordinary dreams, but rather to convey deeper emotions and elicit greater concern.

Being called

A home-based carer told me that she regularly encountered patients who complained of hearing non-existent voices or spoke of being called from the darkness. Research participants themselves relayed the following dream experiences in this regard:

> I used to hear voices when I slept. I heard people say: 'We want to kill you!' [*Hi lava ku nwi dlaya in Tsonga*]. It was only male voices. There were many men. The voices came from outside. I thought it was witches who wanted to make me mad and turn me into a zombie. (Nomsa Ubisi, aged 35, 2013)

> Sometimes, while I slept it felt as if someone shook me. I opened my eyes but found nobody. Then, when I slept again I heard voices call my name. They would say. 'Willem! Where are you? Come here!' The voices were mixed and belonged to many people. (Willem Phako, 52, 2013)

Another time I dreamed of seven-year-old children. They wore
khaki uniforms and held cell [mobile] phones in their right
hands. I did not know one of them, but I was meant to follow
them. The kids were zombies. They were not living humans.
(Reggie Ngobeni, 48, 2008)

Dreamers themselves suggested that the dreams depicted a situation in which witches called them to a 'second world', a world of
darkness and death. Their assailants also sought to transform the
dreamers into diminutive nocturnal servants or zombies (*ditlotlwane*). The association of people suffering from AIDS-related
diseases with zombies, the quintessential living dead, is well established, as has already been noted. Moreover, in the symbolic code
for interpreting ordinary serious dreams, 'small persons' indicate the
presence of witchcraft. These meanings are most cogently expressed
in Reggie Ngobeni's dream of children with mobile phones, calling
him to follow them.

Weddings and virilocal marriage

In women's narratives, the image of weddings and the theme of
marriage elaborate on the fear of being removed from the familiar
world of one's kin. This fear is most directly expressed by the dream
narrated by Jane Nyalungu in the opening vignette of this chapter
and in Pricilla Nyathi's recollection of the following dream:

I walked along the road to Ludlow. I came upon a large
community hall near a mortuary. I entered and saw a wedding
for white people. The pastor was a black man, and he was talking.
I exited the hall and I saw a car with Indians. They called me to
join them, and whispered, 'Come! Come!' When I entered the
car, they tried to clothe me in a wedding dress. They showed
me the groom, who was an Indian man, and in a loud voice I
screamed 'No!' The people in the hall also came out and shouted
at the Indians. They also screamed 'No'. Then I awoke. I was
covered in sweat. (Pricilla Nyathi, 38, 2014)

Following patri-virilocal marriage rules, which are normative
among Northern Sotho and Tsonga-speaking brides, Pricilla Nyathi
took up residence in the unfamiliar homes of the groom and his
kin. This move resonates not only with those of people captured
by witches, but also with those of sick and dying persons who are
progressively alienated from their loved ones. It is significant that

the wedding hall in Pricilla Nyathi's dream was located next to a mortuary. Pricilla told me that her own marriage to a local man ended disastrously. In 2006, her husband separated from her, and since then he had failed to pay maintenance for their four children. 'I am suffering because of that.' Moreover, Pricilla said that she feared the prospect of marrying an Indian man because Indians are foreigners who are prone to practising witchcraft. 'Maybe a white man is better. Maybe he won't allow me to starve.'

Confronting life-threatening danger

Whereas ordinary serious dreams contained omens of pending misfortune, ARV-induced dreams portrayed direct, unmediated encounters with dangerous life-threatening situations. But none of the narrated dreams referred explicitly to HIV/AIDS. Instead, they seemed to have transposed fears of sickness onto other, more concrete, situations of distress. These ranged from confronting intruders in their homes or witnessing warfare to being engulfed by flames or surrounded by stagnant water.

> Once I did not know if I was asleep or awake. I saw a man and a woman in my room, standing right in front of me. They held a stick [knobkerrie] and wanted to beat me. They do not want to talk ... As they were about to hit me, I opened my eye. Then I realised that it was a dream. (Sidney Phiri, 50, 2013)

> I dreamed I saw someone outside my home, trying to open my window. He was a man – a black man. I could see his image. I thought he was a *tsotsi* [thug]. The next morning, I looked for [foot]prints, but I could not see anything.

> I dreamed I looked up and I saw a large mountain. There were lights from the centre of the mountain. They were red – like traffic lights ... There were also large shiny rocks. They made me afraid. I wanted to evade the light, so I turned around ... and I fled through bushes ... Then suddenly soldiers came towards me. (Betwell Ndlovu, 50, 2013)

> I saw visions of soldiers shooting and fighting in the bush outside my home. There was a war and planes were going up and down to prevent the war. Some flew upside down. Some had people, others did not. There were loud sounds from the guns. (Khensani Nkuna, 40, 2013)

I was walking. Then water blocked my way. The water was
stagnant and did not flow. I could not see the end and I could not
swim across. Then I looked back and there was also water. I could
not return, and I was not going to make it. The water surrounded
me. I stood on a small patch of sand. It was not like sea sand – it
was dry, not wet. (Godfrey Mashile, 36, 2013)

We can see these images as multivocal symbols that unite dispa-
rate levels of experience (Turner 1967: 20–4). Images of invaders in
one's house capture explicit xenophobic fears of the uncontrolled
influx of foreigners into Bushbuckridge, and of the transgression of
domestic space by burglars (Niehaus 2012a). At an implicit level, it
might also be suggestive of fears of viruses invading one's body. My
research assistants reminded me that, in Christian teaching, one's
body is a house of the Lord. Images of soldiers, too, have different
referents. They recall a long history of violence associated with the
government's use of security forces to suppress uprisings against the
apartheid system, and, more recently, service delivery protests and
strikes.[8] It is significant that in biomedical discourses the metaphor
of warfare denotes the interaction of viruses and antibodies (called
masoja or 'soldiers' in Northern Sotho) within the body. Research
participants were regularly exposed to these metaphors during
treatment literacy workshops. Images of red lights suggest arrested
travel, as in traffic lights, and stagnant water suggests infertility and
the end of life.

Aggressive animals

Images of animals recurred in narratives about ARV-induced dreams,
particularly those depicting situations of extreme danger.

I saw elephants come from the bush. They entered the houses.
I saw people crying for help. An elephant chased one person,
and he ran, screaming, 'Joojojojojo!' The elephants caught some
people and trampled them to death. (Nomsa Ubisi, 35, 2013)

I heard voices in the forest. To my surprise, I saw baboons
speaking their own language, like humans. There was lots of food
and the baboons were clothed. They were dressed for a wedding.
The priest was a baboon and the guests were all baboons. I was
not afraid, and I wanted to see the wedding. Suddenly a pool of
water appeared. I did not know how to swim, and I feared the
water. (Pricilla Nyathi, 38, 2014)

There were snakes at my gate and inside my room. They were brownish in colour. Some bit me on my hands, others bit my feet. I trampled on them and I ran outside. (Betty Nyalungu, 43, 2013)

I saw frogs jumping and locusts jumping. I also saw a lizard that wanted to drink water ... I also saw a cow fight another cow ... It happened right here in my house, in my bedroom. (Sidney Phiri, 50, 2013)

Residents of Bushbuckridge associated animals with the 'lower self'. In local knowledge, animals lacked the restraints that culture imposed on conduct, and animal behaviours were purely the product of instinct and desire (both *duma*). This was evident in the tendency to refer derogatively to persons who behaved antisocially by animal names: someone who turned against his or her kin might be called a 'dog'; someone who was stubborn or lazy a 'donkey'; and someone who was crooked in financial matters a 'snake'. Similarly, people associated snake- and ape-like witch familiars, such as the *tokolotši* and *mamlambo*, with a lust for money and unrestrained sexual passion (Niehaus et al. 2001: 147–50).

Through narrating dreams about aggressive animals, dreamers broached emotions of anger, which they suppressed from everyday social intercourse. It is noteworthy that during interviews research participants avoided any reference to how, and by whom, they had been infected with HIV. Dream narratives seem to provide an indirect outlet for these tensions. Nomsa Ubisi, the dreamer of vicious elephants, lived with her husband, who, in all likelihood, had infected her with HIV. His surname, Ndlovu, is Setswati for elephant. Other details in these dreams also seem to express disguised fears. Locusts and frogs appear in biblical plagues, and lizards are associated with witchcraft. Villagers believed that witches implanted small reptiles, such as lizards, inside their victims' bodies, to consume their flesh and blood. In the narrated dreams, animals of the forest intruded into village settlements and breached the categorical distinction between nature and culture. This theme is expressed most cogently in Pricilla Nyathi's dream about the wedding of baboons.

Dying and death

In ARV-induced dreams, encounters with death are most apparent in the figures of corpses, skeletons, coffins and graveyards, and in the theme of funerals.

I sometimes dreamed that I was at a funeral. I saw many cars taking a coffin to the grave. (John Mathebula, 54, 2013)

A hearse came towards me, carrying people in coffins. The undertaker stopped the hearse and asked me, 'Come and see the corpses.' When I looked, I saw my dead relatives. They were my elder brother, my sister, and my sister's daughter, who had died long ago. I collapsed of grief. (Dora Mbetse, 38, 2013)

I saw a skeleton and I was scared. The skeleton stood inside my house. It was talking, and its mouth was moving as it spoke … There were also coffins in my home. They were not for me. They were for other people. There were so many coffins in my room. It looked like a mortuary. All the coffins were empty. (Sara Khosa, 35, 2013)

I dreamed that corpses lay scattered on the ground and on the streets. I trampled over the corpses. There were so many, but I could not recognise any of them. It seemed as if someone had killed these people. (Rose Mohlala, 43, 2013)

As we have seen, in Impalahoek there is a well-established equation of HIV/AIDS with death, and persons with AIDS are commonly represented as 'living corpses' who are 'dead before dying'. Years of experiencing the deaths and attending the funerals of kin and neighbours who suffered from AIDS-related diseases reinforced these equations and representations. This is most dramatically apparent in Reggie Ngobeni's accounts of how he witnessed fellow patients die in the tuberculosis ward during 2006 (see Chapter 5). By narrating the dreams noted above, research participants broached the emotionally overwhelming topic of death. It is notable that dreams portrayed the deaths of others. Through time, people's positive responses to HAART and a diminution in the deaths from AIDS-related diseases have generated a new set of concerns, centred on the burden – and perhaps also the guilt – of survivors. Dora Mbetse spoke of the death of her brother, who refused to test for HIV antibodies, two years prior to our interview; and Rose Mohlala referred to the death of her sister, whose three children she cared for, in 2006.

Entering a second world

Dreams of being suspended at height or wandering in another world were also prominent. The emotions associated with such dreams were ambiguous and unclear: they seemed to provoke great anxiety, but sometimes also the desire to enter this 'second world'.

> In my first dream, I found myself standing on top of a very high bridge. I did not know how I got there. There was a rope going down and I descended using the rope, but I could not reach the bottom ... I could not go forward and I could not go backward. It was light, and I could see down there. I could see trees on the ground, but I could not see underneath the trees. (Eric Mnisi, 35, 2013)

> In my dreams, I saw a strange place. There were no houses, but I saw people herding animals. I also saw sheep and green grass. It was a very nice place. I admired it and wished to go there. I tried to get to the people, but could not reach them. Maybe it was heaven. (Godfrey Mashile, 36, 2013)

> Sometimes I found myself on a very high place. I saw myself on a mountain and looked down. I looked from the ridge and saw that it was dark and very deep. I was so scared I would fall. I would sleep close to my husband. (Nomsa Ubisi, 35, 2013)

> I saw myself walking in another country. I did not know where I was. It was not South Africa. I did not know how I got there and I did not know which direction to take. (Richard Mashego, 45, 2013)

The dreams of being suspended on bridges or on mountains, between earth and sky, convey feelings of being in a liminal space outside or beyond ordinary social life (Turner 1967: 94–113). This seems to resonate with being in an anomalous position between sickness and health, marked by fears about the sustainability of HAART, but also by hopes of recovery, couched in religious images of resurrection and salvation. In some dreams, the idea of another world appears as heaven, conceptualised in distinctly Christian terms. Speakers of Northern Sotho sometimes used the word *godimo*, which literally means 'towards God' (*Modimo*), to refer to heights. This meaning is evident in the notion that mountains are quiet places of contemplation, close to God, where Christians pray in times of distress, and where they fast in a search for spiritual renewal (Sundkler 1961: 334).

Visitations by the deceased

As in the case of ordinary serious dreams, visitations by deceased persons in ARV-induced dreams provoked a great deal of interest and discussion. The deceased persons included grandparents, parents, spouses, siblings and children, who might or might not be invoked as ancestors. The deceased were more commonly maternal kin, with whom the dreamer had tender and caring relations, rather than paternal kin, who demanded obedience and respect.

> I saw dead people, those who had passed away long ago. My son, my mother, my father and my grandfather stood in front of me. In real life they are all dead. They did not say anything. They only stood in my room. They walked around where I was sleeping. In my dream, they were naked, all of them. (Nomsa Ubisi, 35, 2013)

> In my dream, I played with my cousin. We were skipping rope. My wife [who is deceased] came to me and said, 'Can't you see it is late! Let's go home!' Then she took me by the hand. (Petros Maunye, 43, 2013)

> I saw my deceased mother's face – not her body, only her face. She told me that everything will be alright. (Betty Mohlala, 28, 2013)

> My grandmother came to me. She came into my room, folded her arms and said, 'You're going to be better!' She was dressed in a long white dress. She looked at me and said: 'You're going to be fine. Don't worry.' (Rose Mohlala, 43, 2013)

Unlike in ordinary serious dreams, the deceased relatives did not indicate their desires, nor issue specific commands. Instead, they were a comforting presence who took the deceased by the hand, reassured them, and promised them that they would recover. The dreams were nonetheless ambiguous. It is unclear whether the deceased simply aided the dreamers' recovery, or else welcomed them to a second world.

The dream below, narrated by John Mathebula, contains more explicit Christian imagery to relay the theme of rescue, and refers to the Holy Spirit rather than the ancestors.

> I dreamed that I was inside a coffin, and that four men carried me towards the cemetery. The men had already dug my grave and they lowered my coffin into the grave. I cried for help and

I hit the inside of the coffin with my fists. Just before my coffin touched the ground, a strong wind came and pushed it from the grave. The men now tied the coffin with ropes and tried to lower it a second time, but the wind again pushed it from the grave. I heard voices saying, 'This man does not want to die! We failed to bury him!' The third time they used a machine from the morgue to lower my coffin. But at the same level the wind pushed the coffin out. Now I was free, and I ran away. The men followed me. But the wind blew me free and put me on level ground. Then I heard another voice, saying, 'My son! I've rescued you! Pray for seven days!' When I woke I touched my chest: I felt my heart pumping very fast. (John Mathebula, 54, 2013)

John Mathebula offered his own interpretation of elements of the dream. He suggested that the four men might have been witches who were envious of his skills as a builder. During the initial stages of his sickness, he said, he believed that he had been a victim of witchcraft. He also suggested that it was God who sent the wind and spoke to him. 'It was a huge voice,' John said. 'An echo followed the words after they were spoken.' In Northern Sotho, the term 'wind' (*moya*) has a broad frame of reference and denotes 'breath', 'spirit' and 'soul'. He drew a definite parallel between religious salvation, as expressed in his dream, and the physical experience of healing.[9]

The sequences of ARV-induced dreams

Thus far, I have shown that a consideration of the figures and themes in narrated ARV-induced dreams offers a unique insight into the deep personal feelings of dreamers, their anxieties about their sickness, and their hopes of healing. However, it is also possible to go beyond an identification of the figures and themes in these dreams (Mageo 2006) and consider the relations between them, and the sequence in which they are told (Kuper 1983).

During interviews, research participants narrated an average of five different ARV-induced dreams, and the temporal sequence in which they were told seems to depict a journey from sickness to near death to renewed life. Dreams of dissociation from everyday life were followed by dreams of confronting life-threatening situations and death; entering a 'second world'; and finally being comforted or saved by mystical forces of good. For many research participants, the journey attested to the mystical powers of HAART.

During 2008 and 2009, research assistants and I interviewed May Mokoena, one of the first AIDS awareness activists in Impala-hoek (see Chapter 3), about his experiences of sickness and therapy. Although May was extremely knowledgeable about biomedical narratives of HIV, AIDS and HAART, he, too, was keen to tell us about the content of his dreams. May said that during 2002 he developed severe gonorrhoea, followed by herpes and shingles. By 2005 his girlfriend had deserted him, and May's health deteriorated to such an extent that he virtually became bedridden. At the zenith of his sickness, May was compelled to wear nappies and begged neighbours to cook for him. In 2006, May tested positive for HIV antibodies, at which time he claimed to have registered a CD4 count of only 34, and began HAART.

The sequence of May's dreams was typical of the narratives that we recorded. His dreams were vivid, and although the theme of dissociation from everyday life was less prominent, the theme of reassurance was over-elaborated. May's first ARV-induced dreams were of being poisoned, witnessing the deaths of others, and attending the funeral of a friend.

> In my very first dream I saw someone – she was a woman;
> I think she was my paternal grandmother – giving me herbs.
> In my dream, I immediately started to be sick. I vomited, I had
> diarrhoea, and sores appeared all over my body. I also started
> to be mentally disturbed.
>   In other dreams, I saw people dying in motor-vehicle
> accidents. Then I found myself walking by a graveyard. I saw
> people burying my friend, who is still alive in real life. In the
> morning, I woke up and started to cry. (May Mokoena, 35, 2009)

In these dreams, May's experience of being poisoned by a woman and his relocation to a mysterious graveyard corresponded with his actual experience of being infected with HIV and with the rapid deterioration of his health. His symptoms of poisoning in his dream were almost identical to those of AIDS-related sicknesses.

In May's next dreams his house was on fire, and his sister, who had died from AIDS-related diseases the previous year, rescued him and reunited him with his former girlfriend, who had deserted him when he became ill.

> I dreamed that my house was on fire. My house was burning
> and everything inside my house was burning, even my bed. Then

my deceased sister arrived. She said, 'I have come to help.' ...
She and her friends came with buckets full of water and they
managed to extinguish the fire.

My sister came to help me a second time. This time she asked
me, 'Where is your wife? Where is your girlfriend?' I told her,
'We're no longer staying together!' Then my sister fetched my
wife and brought her back to me. (May Mokoena, 35, 2009)

May's third dream also dovetails with his experience of sickness. The image of a house on fire seems to be a metaphor for a
body with fever. In Northern Sotho, the term *fiša* (heat) denotes
both pollution and afflictions related to the transgression of taboos
(Hammond-Tooke 1981: 140–3). But May's third and fourth dreams
predict healing (the dousing of the flames by water) and reintegration into social life (the return of his girlfriend). His deceased sister,
although young, appears as an ancestor-like figure who is the agent
of transformation.

May described his final dream, which occurred at a time when he
was severely sick and contemplated committing suicide, as a truly
mystical experience.

I had this dream at midnight. I'll never forget it in all my life.
I lay in my bed. There was no roof on top of the house. It was
only the blue sky. Then my grandmother came from the sky. She
came in the form of an angel. She wore a white cloth, had wings,
and spoke to me. She stood on top [of the bed], raised her hands
and said, 'Son! You'll never die! You'll survive! So, please, go and
preach the gospel!' Then, after a few minutes, she disappeared
into the blue sky. (May Mokoena, 35, 2009)

This ARV-induced dream resembles both the serious dreams
diviners interpret as a calling to their profession and the 'conversion
dreams' Christians narrate during church services. It expresses the
themes of salvation, forgiveness and reunion. May told me that it
was his grandmother, the same person who had poisoned him in
his first dream, who saved him in the final dream. 'In the dream,'
he remarked, 'she came to apologise'. May narrated the later dream
to a pastor of his church, and the pastor suggested that the figure
of his grandmother might have been 'an angel from God'. He and
other research participants who experienced similar dreams noted a
curious correspondence between HAART and the mystical appearance of benevolent spiritual agents. May did not suggest that ARVs

caused ancestors and angels to take an interest in distressed users, but rather that ARV-induced dreams somehow created a portal through which they could manifest themselves to the dreamer.

The journey depicted by the sequence of ARV-induced dreams resonates with the dreamer's experiences of sickness, dissociation from everyday social intercourse, and hopes of recovery and social reintegration. Like the songs and chants of the South American shaman described by Lévi-Strauss (1963), the sequence of dreams orders chaotic sensations and locates them within a meaningful conceptual and discursive framework. They give shape and form to the innermost feelings, anxieties and hopes of persons living with AIDS.

Research participants portrayed the journey, as depicted through the sequence of ARV-induced dreams, as frightening and dangerous, but ultimately as an empowering experience. Undertaking the journey required courage and endurance. Reggie Ngobeni said that he was petrified of the dreams that the tablets gave him. 'Each time the sun set,' he said, 'I used to shiver.' Yet it is through confronting danger and death that the dreamers displayed self-mastery and achieved personal transformation. Livingston (2012) argues that, in Southern Africa, forbearance of pain, both in circumcision lodges and in birthing huts, is essential to growth and to the making of adults. This perception coincides with the Christian concept (shared to some extent by political movements) that suffering is a prerequisite for salvation (and also for the attainment of political liberation). Danger and pain 'battle-hardened' those people who endured them (Heald 1986). This logic is evident in the status of widows in Impalahoek. Having experienced the death of a spouse, widows were deemed to have acquired a certain level of immunity against the pollution of death. Only widows could undertake certain tasks at funerals, such as cleansing corpses, comforting the bereaved, and burning the mourning attire of other widows who had recently been released from a state of mourning.

Although frightening, ARV-induced dreams nonetheless diluted the emotionally overwhelming experience of AIDS-related sicknesses. The dreams depicted dreamers confronting intruders and heights, rather than their own decomposing bodies, and predators rather than their own lovers and spouses, who had infected them with HIV. They externalised death by showing the corpses of others, or placed death in a positive light by showing dreamers receiving money, roaming in a fertile 'second world', or being reunited with deceased kin.

The experience of recovery and healing was, nonetheless, uneven. Three research participants who claimed to have faithfully adhered to HAART initially recovered from opportunistic infections, but then succumbed to death. Health workers described these setbacks as being due to drug-resistant tuberculosis. Another HAART user, who was pregnant and severely ill in 2012, lost her baby but fully regained her own health. Godfrey Mashile and May Mokoena made the most dramatic recoveries. Godfrey's weight almost doubled, from 34 to 63 kilograms, in less than a year, and May's CD4 count climbed from 34 in 2005 to 781 in 2007. Five research participants said that a remarkable aspect of their recovery was that they had gained certain mystical powers and were now able to predict and foretell the occurrence of future events through dreams. This is evident in the opening vignette of Jane Nyalungu, who claimed that ARV-induced dreams had strengthened her divinatory abilities. Likewise, May Mokoena remarked: 'Now [since his recovery], if I dream of something it will happen.' He said that whenever he dreamed of gravel roads, buses, cars or a feast, there would be a funeral. Doris Malebe, another research participant who received HAART, relayed that she, too, gained the gift of prophecy. A recent dream, she said, foretold the death of a distant cousin. 'Being sick has given me special power.'[10]

Conclusions

The transnational distribution of ARVs and universal modes of treating HIV/AIDS have not brought about unitary 'regimes of values' nor a 'thickening hegemony' of biomedical discourses (Butt 2011: 319). Rather, the circulation or flow of ARVs has given rise to 'enclavings' in which producers, nationalist elites, clinicians, community-based health workers and consumers might impose different meanings on them (Van der Geest et al. 1996). Participants in this study have not subscribed to the controversial view of President Mbeki and his Health Ministry that ARVs are lethally toxic and adversely affect the life course of people with AIDS. They have, however, deployed a far broader perspective than the biomedical one, and have used criteria that are very different from biochemical effects to evaluate their efficacy. Research participants saw ARVs in the context of a broader 'health world', a comprehensive *telos* of well-being that refers not merely to the physical integrity of the body but also to the person's standing in relation to other social actors and spiritual agencies (Germond and Cochrane 2010).

In Impalahoek, vivid dreams were not simply a side effect of medication; they were integral to the workings of HAART (Etkin

1992). This understanding is contiguous with existing ideas about the workings of herbal medicines and about the significance of serious dreams. These ideas constitute a template for interpreting the meanings of ARV-induced dreams. Despite their frightening and sometimes dreadful content, the dreams have by no means impeded adherence to HAART. But more than this, an analysis of the sequence of ARV-induced dreams points to a belief in the transformative effect of medication. Dreams of danger battle-harden dreamers against suffering, and dreams of corpses immunise them against the pollution of death. These are followed by dreams that seem to provide a portal for spiritual agencies – such as the ancestors and the Holy Spirit – to assist and comfort persons living with AIDS. For these reasons, ARVs are deemed to possess 'mystical efficacy' (Van der Geest et al. 1996: 169).

To comprehend the relationship of ARV-induced dreams to everyday life, we can turn once more to Lévi-Strauss's (1963) analysis of the South American *cuna* ritual. He argues that the work of the shaman – who conducts this ritual – resembles that of the psychoanalyst. But there is one difference: whereas the shaman speaks and relays a myth, the psychoanalyst merely listens and assists the patient to construct her or his own myth, drawing on elements from the past (ibid.: 204). In these terms, ARV-induced dreams speak to the dreamers, by enabling them to conceptualise and reflect on aspects of their experience and consciousness that might otherwise be inaccessible. But dreamers also speak through these dreams to others and articulate what may otherwise be unsayable.

7
Care

On 19 August 2014, I visited the Ekuruleni ('Safe Haven' in Tsonga) Centre for Orphans and Vulnerable Children. The construction of the centre in a village behind Tintswalo hospital was a unique achievement that involved cooperation by a former nurse, Betty Ngwenya, home-based carers, a head teacher who was also an acting chief, and American-based charities. The activists believed that such a centre would address a most urgent need arising from the HIV/AIDS pandemic. In 2010, the records of schools in the vicinity showed that 592 learners had lost one or both parents (probably largely due to AIDS-related diseases) or had parents who were desperately ill and were receiving home-based care. Betty Ngwenya, the director of Ekuruleni, told me: 'There is nothing as bitter as to be without a parent, especially a mother.'

Betty and her colleagues established a board of trustees and started raising funds from Christian organisations, such as Seeds of Life, and from the social responsibility departments of businesses such as Telkom, Polar Air and Nedbank. They then commissioned the well-known architect Nina Cohen, who designed the Nelson Mandela Museum in Johannesburg, to draw up building plans. The centre officially opened in 2012, and immediately admitted 100 children between the ages of five and 18. (Their number had grown to 153 by 2004, when I visited the centre.) Betty explained to me that all users had to be registered. 'This is because we are responsible for them.' The centre employed a staff of 20 young women who received stipends from the government's Department of Social Development. The staff prepared breakfast and lunch for all the children at weekends and during holidays, but only one meal on ordinary school days, and offered a wide range of activities to prepare them for the future. These included permaculture, gardening, art and drama, computer literacy, football, netball and volleyball. They also allocated tasks such as cleaning to the children. There were large ablution blocks, where children could wash themselves and their clothes, and a 'skills development centre' that housed a library and desks, where the older learners could do their homework. Betty was satisfied that the children were well cared for. She said that many children had learned to speak English and observed that they were extremely happy when playing games such as Sarafina.[1] Betty remarked: 'Some come here with little self-esteem and with sores all over their bodies, but now have a good appearance.' In the future, Betty said, the board of trustees wished to secure long-term funding and improve facilities so that they could also admit younger children.

These achievements are impressive. Here, in a part of the world where development projects seldom pay dividends (Ferguson 1990), was a centre that worked well and seemed to be responsive to local need. But I had a nagging question: 'Where are the sleeping quarters?' Betty replied that there were none. The board had planned to build accommodation for 38 children but encountered stiff opposition. 'The community argued that we should not isolate children from their families.' Therefore, the centre only cared for the children from the morning, or from the period after school, until family members came to fetch them in the early evening. Moreover, she said, their parents and guardians gave regular input into the management of Ekuruleni.

My visit to the Ekuruleni Centre highlighted two crucial issues. First, it showed a divergence of the concerns of biopolitical theorists and those of local activists. Whereas the former focus more narrowly on sick people, their needs, rights and responsibilities, Betty Ngwenya and her colleagues displayed broader concerns that incorporated the plight of certain survivors of the pandemic. The latter concern was shared by commentators who projected that the AIDS pandemic might create as many as 4.6 million orphans in South Africa by 2013 (Bray 2003: 408). Such a projection provoked intense fears of an impending crisis of homeless children who would live without adult care, and of a concomitant rise in disorder and crime. Globally, fundraisers have used the concept of 'AIDS orphans', rhetorically, to secure access to much-needed resources (Bornstein 2001; Meintjes and Griese 2006). Moreover, in South Africa, welfare has been organised according to social vulnerability rather than biology, as was the case in the Ukraine after the Chernobyl catastrophe (Petryna 2002: 115–48). Here, government has been more prominent in the distribution of non-contributory social benefits, via non-market cash payments, than in the provision of HIV/AIDS clinics and treatment. Such benefits included child support grants of R300 (£18) per child per month in 2014 and child foster grants of R920 (£56) per child per month that were introduced to meet post-apartheid expectations and in response to the emergence of vast numbers of AIDS orphans (Ferguson 2015).

Second, my visit showed the resilience of existing kinship structures. In Impalahoek, hardly any AIDS orphans lived on the streets or in child-headed households, without adult care. Instead, they continued to remain part of broader networks of kinship and relatedness and were regularly cared for by surviving parents and other kin. As such, the centre played a complementary rather than supplementary role in the provision of childcare. As Meintjes and Griese (2006) argue, the experience of orphan-hood is far from uniform and varies by social and cultural context. It is thus important to recognise caregivers who are still alive, and to distinguish between fatherless, motherless, and wholly parentless children. They contend that a focus on orphans may well obscure an understanding of the multiple ways in which AIDS affects children who live in situations of poverty. Though prioritised for relief, orphans might well live better lives than many vulnerable children with parents (ibid.).

In line with these observations, my aim in this chapter is to explore the complex subtleties of social relations in the domestic settings of Impalahoek that have enabled care for AIDS orphans. In so doing, I build on the insights of previous studies that have drawn attention to creative improvisations by residents of Southern African, first in response to the system of labour migration, which separated husbands from their wives and fathers from sons and daughters,[2] and second in response to the pandemic of AIDS-related deaths. In the case of Lesotho, Ansell and van Blerk (2004) assert that the extraordinary adaptability of households has facilitated childcare. Here, surviving household members have deployed the established practice of dispersing dependants to cope with the devastating impact of AIDS deaths.[3] In 1992, before the advent of the pandemic, 22 per cent of households in Lesotho contained children who were not offspring of the household head. By 1999, this percentage had risen to 33 per cent (ibid.: 679). Ansell and van Blerk (ibid.) argue that, contrary to customary law, which posits that the children of deceased parents should remain in the paternal line, matrilineal kin frequently took care of orphans. Concerns such as the capacity of households to accommodate the children and the potential contributions that children could make to domestic and agricultural work often outweighed legal conventions (ibid.: 689). In Mokhotlong, Lesotho, Block (2014) also discerns a disjuncture between 'official' and 'practical' kinship. Despite the official model of patrilineal descent, 75 per cent of orphans resided with maternal kin such as grandmothers. This is because, during illness, women frequently returned to their natal homes with their children. Maternal caregivers argued that the children could not affiliate to the paternal line because their fathers had not completed bridewealth payments.

In another study of the care of AIDS orphans, in Magangan-gozi, KwaZulu-Natal, Henderson (2006) argues that the children of deceased parents drew on 'layered repertoires of relatedness' to reposition themselves in kinship networks and create new social bonds. They moved between the homes of different kin, initiated ties with neighbours by ploughing their fields, and contracted informal marriages. These strategies were not seamless, but they generally secured children's survival (ibid.).

While I acknowledge the theme of improvisation, the aim of this chapter diverges from the studies noted above by investigating the guardianship of AIDS orphans in Impalahoek in the light of contemporary Northern Sotho and Shangaan models of kinship. I contend that childcare arrangements are an outcome of complex negotiations not simply within households, but also within broader kinship networks. In poorer residential areas such as Impalahoek, households are seldom economically independent, and they do not constitute self-evident units of analysis (Segalen 1984). In these contexts, kinship is a potentially valuable template for social organ-isation, and a resource for mutual aid. This has been especially pertinent during the HIV/AIDS pandemic. Whereas AIDS-related diseases and deaths weakened relations built on marriage and affinity (see Chapter 3), they have led to a renewed focus on rela-tions of consanguinity. Unlike Block (2014), I do not discern any disjuncture between official and practical kinship. This is largely because Northern Sotho and Shangaan models of kinship posit several alternative guardians and carers, among both paternal and maternal kin. An important principle of both models is the diffusion of parenthood – or at least of parental work – among the father's and mother's siblings. In recognising a child's aunts and uncles as complementary and substitute parents, I suggest, these models leave considerable room for manoeuvre and choice. Moreover, I demon-strate that in contemporary South Africa, state-sponsored welfare grants have had a powerful effect on the care and guardianship of AIDS orphans. As in the case of Lesotho, I detect a shift towards guardianship by maternal kin, particularly by the mother's sister and mother's mother (Ansell and van Blerk 2004; Block 2014). But I do not see this shift as merely an outcome of the vagaries of marriage: it is also due to women's relative ease of access to child maintenance and foster grants.

Kinship and the diffusion of parenthood

Northern Sotho and Shangaan kinship models, as described by adult research participants during fieldwork, shared certain noteworthy features.[4] In both cases, social organisation was supposed to be patrilineal. After a husband had paid the initial instalment of bridewealth, a newly married couple was expected to take up residence in the hamlet (*motse*) of his parents. Here, they remained for a few years before establishing their own, independent, household. Children adopted their father's surname and his sons inherited his cattle and estate.

Nonetheless, both paternal and maternal kin were important to a child's upbringing. Grandparents (*kokwane*) on both sides were expected to sustain affectionate relations with their grandchildren and to spoil rather than discipline them. They were permitted to indulge in joking with their grandchildren, a practice that marks an ambiguous disjunction and conjunction of status. Despite belonging to different generations, grandparents and grandchildren are both seen to be asexual and dependent (Radcliffe-Brown 1952b; Stadler 1994: 89).

The father (*tate*) was, conceptually, the authoritative 'owner of the hamlet' (*mong wa motse*). He settled disputes, enclosed and guarded its borders, and represented it to the outside word. The male space within the hamlet comprised a shaded area near the entrance, called *kgôrô* (which literally means 'gate' or 'court'). A father named his children and thereby bestowed their social identity. He was also expected to discipline them and provided for their material needs.

Both Northern Sotho and Shangaan kinship models were premised on the 'equivalence of siblings' (Radcliffe-Brown 1950), and paternal responsibilities were diffused among the father, his brothers and his sisters. The father's brothers were expected to substitute for him and, in his absence, settle disputes within his household and provide food for his dependants. The father's brothers were the first to be informed when a girl became pregnant out of wedlock, or when any child was sick, and were expected to make appropriate arrangements. However, there were some distinctions between elder and junior brothers. The father's older brother (*ramogolo*; literally 'big father') ideally commanded the greatest respect and acted as a kind of genealogist who informed children about their ancestors and kin. The younger brother (*rangwane*, or 'small father') was expected to negotiate bridewealth payments. The father's sister (*rakgadi*) should also act with authority, which was uncharacteristic for a woman. In ritual contexts, she was perceived as senior to her brothers, and her children were senior to theirs. This was because, in the past, brothers relied on cattle from the marriages of their sisters for bridewealth, and seniority accrued to the giver of cattle. She was expected to recite the family's praise poem on occasions such as weddings, and to invoke the father's ancestors (*badimo*) in times of distress. It was also incumbent on her to advise nephews and nieces on marriage, to ensure that all bridewealth was paid, and to instruct young wives on how they should behave at the home of their in-laws. The father's siblings had collective responsibility for arranging the funerals of his children, should they die unexpectedly at an early age.

As in the case of patrilineal models of social organisation elsewhere, wives retained membership of the descent groups of their fathers and were still addressed by their maiden surnames. Metaphorically, bridewealth only transferred rights over a woman's body to her affines: her head remained the property of her agnates. Her parents and siblings regularly visited her and sustained an active interest in the welfare of her children. Her sisters helped to bathe and feed her babies, and carried them on their backs. They taught her older children household chores, such as fetching wood and water, cleaning, cooking, and washing clothes. Ideally, the older sister (*mmamogolo* or 'big mother'), like the grandmother, was a font of wisdom about tradition and customs. The younger sister (*mangwane* or 'small mother') taught the girls personal hygiene and informed them about sexual matters. She could also assist in bridewealth negotiations.

Traditionally, the mother's brother (*malome*)[5] was expected to act as guardian (*mohlokomedi*) to his sister's children (Radcliffe-Brown 1952a). He was expected to arrange therapy when they were sick, to discipline them when they disobeyed their mother, and to assume a leading role in arranging their funerals, should they die young. His wife (*mmamalume*) was obliged to assist him in these tasks. Generally, the relation between maternal uncle and his sister's children should be intimate, open and supportive. Boys should feel comfortable enough to discuss sensitive matters with him. In terms of Shangaan kinship models, a nephew was permitted to take food from his mother's brother's home without asking for permission. (This practice was called *didela*.) The mother's brother, in turn, should defend the children in times of trouble, such as when they were accused of witchcraft. In ritual contexts, the mother's brother was seen to be junior to his nephews, and his wife was junior to his nieces. The nephews should taste the first fruit of the season before him. My research assistant, who was Northern Sotho, always spoke Tsonga to his nephew, whose father was Shangaan. 'This is respect [*hlompa*],' he said.

Both Northern Sotho and Shangaan kinship models required intimate, close and supportive relations between siblings, and deemed sibling rivalry to be scandalous. Older siblings were obliged to care for younger ones. This was evident in 'socialisation by peers' (Mayer and Mayer 1970) and in the practice of sibling guardianship (called *rufa* in Northern Sotho). Sometimes a newly married couple was obliged to take care of a younger sibling of the husband: the husband paid for his sibling's education and his wife cooked for him or her and washed clothes his or her clothes.

A key difference in Northern Sotho and Shangaan models pertained to cousins. In Northern Sotho, people called parallel cousins (children of the MZ or FB)[6] by the same terms as siblings (*ngwanešo* when of the same sex, or *kgaetsedi* when of the opposite sex); but they called cross-cousins (children of the MB or FZ) *motswala* (a term with no age or sex distinctions). Cross-cousins were not 'of the same blood' and were permitted – and even encouraged – to have sexual intercourse and marry. Here, the marital strategy was based on preserving the lineage's integrity and on ensuring the return of bridewealth across generations. Cross-cousins also enjoyed a relationship that permitted joking and disrespect, to diffuse any tensions between them (Radcliffe-Brown 1952b).

In Tsonga, too, people also called parallel cousins by the same name as siblings (*buti* for male and *tate* for female). But maternal cross-cousins (MBd or MBs) were called *manana* ('mother') and *malume* ('mother's brother'), and paternal cross-cousins (FZd or FZs) *n'wana* ('son') and *n'wana wa wanhwana* ('daughter'). The significance of these terms appears when we read them in conjunction with exogamy rules. In the Shangaan model, unlike Northern Sotho one, cross-cousins are not allowed to have sex or marry, but a young woman is entitled to marry her father's sister's husband as a second wife (Kuper 1982). This practice extends and further cements marriage alliances (Webster 1977: 193). It also suggests a caring, maternal, relationship between cross-cousins.

At the time of fieldwork, these kinship models were largely models *for* rather than models *of* conduct (Geertz 1973), and they described ideal rather than real states of affairs. During the 2000s, bridewealth exchanges had diminished, patrilocal residence was less common, and cross-cousin marriage had almost entirely disappeared. There were also profound changes in inheritance. Since the

1960s, the last-born son and his wife had been expected to occupy the home of his parents. This did not amount to preferential treatment, because it was incumbent on him and his wife to care for the ageing parents (James 1987). But the nomenclature of the classificatory kinship models described above attained renewed significance in the context of the migrant labour system. These set out broad, polyvalent paternal obligations, predicated on blood, descent and marriage. Ideally, the work of grandparents, uncles, aunts, older siblings and even cousins complemented that of the mother and father, and ensured that parenthood assumed plural rather than singular forms.

Such indeterminacy accords formal Northern Sotho and Shangaan kinship models with special resilience when confronting the formidable challenges of childcare. During 1991, at the very start of the HIV/AIDS pandemic, Eliazaar Mohlala and I conducted a social survey of 87 households. The results indicated that only 42.0 per cent of children under 18 (191 of 455) physically resided in the same household as their parents: 46.6 per cent (212) lived without their fathers, 3.3 per cent (15) without mothers, and 8.1 per cent (37) without both parents. Many parents were at work in South Africa's centres of mining and industry, their absence from home being a prerequisite to their children's survival. But there were also cases of severe impoverishment, separation, divorce and death within the parental generation. In some situations, parents dispersed their children to the homes of adult relatives who were in a better position to care for them (Spiegel 1986). In others, children resided in extended households that included the remaining parent, paternal grandparents, uncles and aunts, siblings and parallel cousins.

The diffusion of parental obligations enabled various categories of kin to act as guardians for orphans. There were no fewer than 47 orphans in the sampled households: 21 (45 per cent) resided solely with their surviving parent and with uterine siblings; five (10 per cent) with paternal kin such as grandparents and the father's siblings; and 21 (45 per cent) with maternal kin, such as grandparents and the mother's siblings. In situations where a husband who had paid full bridewealth had died, it was ideally incumbent upon his brother to assume full conjugal and paternal responsibilities on his behalf (an institution called the levirate in kinship terminology). Where a married woman had died, her younger sister – or, in the case of Shangaans, her brother's daughter – could assume her responsibilities as wife and mother (the sororate). But with growing emphasis on individual choice in marriage partners (Thomas 2009), and with a concomitant decrease in arranged marriages and in bridewealth transfers, these arrangements have become uncommon.

An alternative and increasingly common option was for maternal kin to assume responsibility for the guardianship of orphans. 'Long ago,' said a middle-aged Shangaan man, 'it [the guardian] had to be the mother's brother [*malume*].' This arrangement was most appropriate where the father still owed bridewealth. But one research participant argued that the mother's brother was the proper guardian even when the father had paid all the bridewealth. 'The father,' he argued, 'might remarry and his second wife will trouble the children because they are not hers.' Mabetha Mapayile told me that in 1969 his sister, Lilian, and her two sons were in desperate financial trouble after her husband, who was a bus driver, died tragically in a road accident. The husband's employer promised to help Lilian out financially, but only twice deposited groceries at her home. Lilian subsequently secured employment as a farm labourer near White River but was unable to take her children with her. Mabetha, who was a teacher, took care of Lilian's youngest son, and his brother, Timothy, who was a traffic policeman, took the oldest. Only during the early 1980s, when both boys were in high school, did they return to their mother's home. By now she earned a living by selling fruit and vegetables from home, and by working as a Christian healer. Mabetha considered his efforts to be part of his social obligation and never referred to the status of Lilian's affines. Such cases were not exceptional. Where an unmarried mother was deceased, her mother or a sister could also act as the primary guardian.

HIV/AIDS and marriage

A diminution in the frequency and stability of marriage during the 1990s had a direct impact on the status of children and, more specifically, of AIDS orphans. Traditionally, parents helped sons pay bridewealth, which was set at ten cows for a Northern Sotho bride, and 13 cows for a Shangaan bride. But as households lost their cattle – due to the devastating epizootic of 1958 and the imposition of stock limitations by government – young men started to pay their own bridewealth in cash. Moreover, the value of bridewealth was no longer standard, but depended on the bride's educational qualifications. In 26 marriages recorded in another Bushbuckridge village during the 1980s and early 1990s, the value of bridewealth varied from R120 for a young woman with no formal schooling to R12,000 for a bride with a nursing diploma (Stadler 1994).

In this changing context, only wealthier businessmen and well-paid employees could afford to pay bridewealth in full and instantly attain the status of husband and father. Ordinary miners and factory workers, who had manifold financial obligations, experienced the payment of bridewealth as a drawn-out process. They usually paid a negotiated initial instalment, in order for the wife to take up residence in their home, and then settled the outstanding debt to her parents over a period of many years. As in the case of Lesotho (see Block 2014), a wife's status was often profoundly liminal, and the affiliation of her children insecure. The system of labour migration also contributed to profound marital disharmony. The separation of husbands from their wives was conducive to extramarital affairs, and young women frequently found it extremely stressful to reside in the home of their in-laws while their husbands were at work (Niehaus et al. 2001: 98–106). Our household survey in 1991, however, revealed high rates of marriage: 64.5 per cent (120 of 186) of adult men and 63.7 per cent (123 of 193) of adult women were married.[7] Seventy-two per cent of children (318 of 439) resided with or belonged to the same household as their fathers.

The next two decades saw a decline in marriage; this can be correlated with job losses resulting from de-industrialisation, with the downscaling of mines and the closure of factories. New employment opportunities in the service sector – for taxi drivers, security guards, shop assistants and game lodge employees – did not compensate for these losses (Niehaus 2006a). Indeed, the percentage of unemployed men in sampled households increased from 16 per cent during 1991 to 48 per cent in 2004. In this context of increased financial hardship, fewer men could afford to pay bridewealth and secure paternity over their children. A survey of the same 87 households, when revisited during 2004, showed that only 48.1 per cent (112 of 233) of adult men and 37.5 per cent (113 of 301) of adult women were married. However, the median age of marriage had not increased.

More children were now born to single mothers. Previously, many fathers had been absent migrant labourers who supported their children financially and saw them occasionally during vacations from work. Now they were more likely to be absent altogether – not only in a *de facto* sense, but also in a *de jure* one. During 2004, only 50.6 per cent (251 of 496) children resided with or belonged to the same household as their fathers. The loss of income derived from remittances sent home by male migrants was offset by a slight increase in women's access to employment, and by a considerable increase in state-instituted social security payments, such as pensions and grants. These grants made a very significant contribution to household income. In 2004, 20 households in our sample (23 per cent) survived solely on social welfare. The absence of fathers also led to increased childcare responsibilities for the mother's siblings and maternal grandparents (Schatz and Ogunmefun 2007: 1391). The mother's brothers often helped financially, while her sisters looked after her children and cooked for them.

The HIV/AIDS pandemic exacerbated conjugal stress and marital breakdown. As we saw in Chapter 3, the discovery that a spouse had been infected with a deadly virus – probably by an extra-marital lover – was the pretext for blame, bitter recriminations and severe conflict. Mfecane (2010) studied the problems faced by 25 HIV-positive men in Bushbuckridge who were using HAART and attending support groups in disclosing their status to their partners. Some decided not to disclose, out of the fear that their wives would desert them and take away their children. Others disclosed only after their wives had promised to remain and care for them should they be HIV-positive. Mfecane found that seven (41 per cent) of the 17 men who did disclose their status were abandoned by their wives. In the ten other cases, their wives remained, feeling obliged to support the men they loved in challenging times (ibid.: 183). My research findings were roughly similar: six (46 per cent) of 13 HIV-positive men and 13 (59 per cent) of 22 HIV-positive women reported that their spouses or partners deserted them when the nature of their sickness became apparent.[8] One research participant, Joseph Khosa, who was married and worked in Gauteng, returned home to his mother after he became desperately ill. Over the next five years, Joseph's wife visited him only once in Impalahoek. Some HIV-positive women recalled that their husbands found new wives, or simply abandoned them. There were also men and women who wished to support their sick partners, but, because not all of the bridewealth had been paid, they were prohibited from being part of the 'therapy management group' (Janzen 1978).

HIV/AIDS and childcare

Parental deaths during the HIV/AIDS pandemic have accorded orphans greater visibility. The Mpumalanga provincial government obliged teachers at all schools to submit regular reports recording the exact numbers of orphans in local schools. One such report stated that, in 2004, 139 out of 1,140 (12 per cent) learners at the Impalahoek primary school were orphaned. Fifty-eight learners were 'maternal', 66 'paternal', and 15 'double' orphans. These calculations approximate the results of the survey of 87 households that Eliazaar Mohlala and I conducted in Impalahoek. During 2004, 12 per cent (59 of 496) children under the age of 18 years were orphans. There seemed to have been a further increase subsequently. During 2009, estimates by the Mpumalanga government placed the total proportion of orphans in the province at 18.7 per cent (Weckesser 2011: 127).

South African government policy has been premised on the assumption that kin and household members, other than parents, can provide appropriate care for AIDS orphans. This was evident when government introduced foster grants to the value of R780 per child, paid each month to adults recognised as the legal guardians of orphans. But successful grant applications required a careful navigation of the state bureaucracy. Potential guardians needed unabridged birth certificates and proper identity documents for the orphaned children, death certificates of their parents, proof of residence letters, and signed affidavits made at the police station. In addition, social workers had to assess the financial needs and suitability of the guardian, and this had to be confirmed by the magistrate. Hence, the grant formalised the status of guardianship.

Residents of Impalahoek were generally opposed to Western-style adoptions. The wealthy owner of a chicken run, who was infertile, was known to have adopted two unrelated children. My research assistants felt that such arrangements were inappropriate and commented that the businessman was on bad terms with his siblings. 'As the black community,' a middle-aged woman told me, 'we are not used to such things.' Some research participants referred to the Northern Sotho saying 'A cows does not lick another cow's calf' (*Kgomo ga e latswe namane ya e ngwe*) to emphasise that non-kin do not provide proper childcare. Others suspected that severe problems would arise when children were not of the same blood as their guardians. For example, unrelated children might disrespect their social parents and insist on knowing who their 'real' mothers and fathers were.

In the opinion of research participants, the most appropriate arrangement was for an adult relative to act as guardian (*mohloko-medi*) for an orphaned child.[9] Table 7.1 shows the various categories of cognatic kin who acted as prime guardians and caretakers of 63 orphans in 22 households. The table shows that only one orphan was cared for by an unrelated person, who was a close friend of her deceased mother. When Aletta Mnisi died from complications arising from AIDS-related diseases, she had been twice divorced and was caring for three children – Lenetta (19) and the twins Grace and Gloria (both 16). Aletta's grandmother and mother assumed guardianship of Lenetta and Grace. Gloria, however, decided to stay with Patricia Namane, a wealthy woman friend of her mother, whose family owned a hotel and bottle store.

Table 7.1 Primary guardians of AIDS orphans, Impalahoek, 2014

Kinship relation	Number	Percentage
Siblings	10	15.9
Father's mother	1	1.6
Father's brother	5	7.9
Father's sister	2	3.2
Father's cousin	1	1.6
Mother's father	3	4.8
Mother's mother	14	22.2
Mother's sister	19	30.2
Mother's brother	7	11
Mother's friend	1	1.6
Total	63	100

Gloria cleaned Patricia's home after school and ran errands for her. This arrangement eased the financial burden of childcare. Patricia and Aletta's relationship had been exceptionally close, and in some ways analogous to kinship (Killick and Desai 2012). The child reportedly reminded Patricia of her deceased friend, and in some ways eased the pain of the loss.

Table 7.1 also depicts a growing shift towards guardianship by maternally related kin, and by women relatives. Ten (16 per cent) orphans were cared for by uterine siblings, nine (14 per cent) by patrilineal kin, and 44 (70 per cent) by maternally related relatives. Here, older notions of kinship and guardianship were reconfigured in the context of current economic concerns, such as economic hardship and access to foster grants.

Patrilineal kin

Despite the proliferation of children born to single mothers, the diminution of bridewealth payments and the virtual disappearance of the levirate, the principle of care by paternal relatives had persisted and continued to be relevant in current circumstances.

Paternal kin tended to act as guardians for orphans when they had sufficient social and financial resources to do so, when they had settled all bridewealth debts, and when the deceased mother had resided with her husband's kin. This was apparent during 2013 and 2014, when the brothers Enos and James Shokane both lost their wives due to AIDS-related diseases. The two brothers were securely married and resided in an extended household with their mother (a pensioner, who had separated from their father), their brother Samson (a police officer, who was married and had two children), and their sister Doris (an unemployed single mother with two children). Enos Shokane operated a relatively successful business that hired out tents for occasions such as funerals, and James was employed in a relatively well-remunerated position in Johannesburg. The deaths of their wives left three maternal orphans between the ages of six and 12 years. In this case, the orphans' paternal kin had sufficient income to care for them and did not wish to separate them from their grandmother and parallel cousins. Despite occasional tensions between the women of the Shokane household over issues such as household budgets in the past, they effectively suppressed all strife to display reluctant solidarity (Bahre 2007) in the face of fatal illness and death.

In one exceptional case, Ben Mokoena asked his cousin (FBs) Henry Mokoena and Henry's first wife, Betty, to be guardians of his 12-year-old daughter, Alusia. During 2002, Ben had lost his wife and was severely ill. When Henry visited him, Ben reportedly asked: 'Should I die, look after my child.' Henry assumed the role of guardian in the belief that the last words of any dying person possessed innate power and could bring severe misfortune should they be disobeyed. He told me of the Northern Sotho proverb: 'What the deceased says must be followed' (*Lentsu le hohu ga a tshelwe*). This arrangement was considered appropriate because Ben was not on good terms with his own household members and more immediate kin. Henry was a senior policeman and his wife, Betty, was infertile and could not have children herself. Alusia assisted them with chores at home and came to address Betty as 'mother' (*mma*). Alusia's child, who was born in 2008, called her 'grandmother' (*kokwane*). Ben's own siblings did not object to this arrangement. His sister occasionally visited Alusia, to provide whatever support she could.

The mother's brother

With growing singleness and broken marriages, attention increasingly focused on the mother's brother (*malume*), whom many see as the traditional guardian of his sister's children. But the mother's brother cared for only seven out of 63 orphans (11 per cent) in the sampled households. We can partially account for this tendency in terms of the reluctance of welfare bureaucrats of the South African Social Security Association to allocate foster grants to men or to unrelated women, such as the mother's brother's wife (*mmamalome*). A social survey of 1,886 grant applications in the Agincourt district of Bushbuckridge during 2002 shows that only 8 (0.4 per cent) applications were made by male relatives, such as fathers and uncles (Twine et al. 2007: 123). One research participant, reflecting on this situation, told me: 'Our government causes trouble. They [presumably social workers] will not give child maintenance and foster money to the *malome*.'

Henry Mokoena and his wife, Betty, told me that in addition to caring for his paternal cousin's daughter, Alusia, they acted as guardians of his sister's four children. Henry's sister and her husband, who had been next-door neighbours, died in 1998 and 1999 respectively. Henry was chosen as guardian because of his status as the mother's brother, his relative prosperity, and the fact that Betty was infertile. 'I do not have my own [children],' she told me, 'therefore I take care of others ... This is God's plan for me.' At the time, the oldest orphan, Robina, who was 15 years of age, and her siblings continued to reside in their deceased mother's home. The children washed themselves and cleaned their own rooms, but Henry paid for all necessities, and Betty cooked for them. Eventually, the household managed to secure a disability grant for the youngest child, who was profoundly deaf. The grant was paid directly to Robina, as his oldest sister. Betty was unhappy about this arrangement and alleged that Robina sometimes misused the grant. To obtain sufficient money for supporting the children, Betty occasionally worked on a nearby fruit farm. During her absence, she sent the youngest boy, who regularly broke things such as glasses and plates at home, and bullied other children in the neighbourhood, to a crèche.

In other cases, the issue of social grants was also a problem. John Nziane told me that he was shaken by the untimely death of his sister and felt a deep moral obligation to become the guardian of her five remaining children. But John could afford to care for only the youngest two children. Social workers had registered the sister of the children's estranged father as legal guardian, and only she was entitled to collect the foster grants. This prompted the oldest three children to take up residence with paternal kin.

However, I heard endless complaints by orphans that their mother's brothers were unwilling to assume their traditional responsibilities as guardian or had failed to provide proper financial support. In an interview, Mary Mogale recalled that, after the death of her unmarried mother and her grandmother in 2007, she and her sister – who were both in their mid-teens – continued to reside in their natal homestead. They had three maternal uncles: a medical doctor in Nelspruit (who was married with three children), a boiler-maker in Johannesburg, and a construction worker in Machadodorp (the latter two were both single). The boilermaker regularly deposited money in their bank account – sometimes up to R1,000 – but he ceased to do so once he married and had his own children. Mary blamed the wives of her maternal uncles.

> Our uncles were okay, but not their wives. They liked us when our mother was still alive, but after she died they showed their true colours. They came between our uncles and us ... Nowadays the *malome*'s wife dominates. He will say: 'My wife does not allow me to take care of my sister's children.'

Apart from pressing financial concerns and the issue of access to foster grants, there were factors intrinsic to concepts of kinship that made wives reluctant to care for the children of their husband's sister. Traditionally, I was told, the relationship between a man's wife and sister was tense. Because a man used cattle from his sister's marriage as bridewealth, his sister claimed seniority over his wife, and her children claimed entitlement to greater privileges than their cousins. Should a man become the guardian of this sister's children, these claims would undermine the vitally important principle of equivalence between siblings. In the case of Northern Sotho households, there was the additional recognition and fear that foster children were entitled to have sex with, and even to marry, a man's biological children. This concern was particularly acute when orphans were poor and were suspected of having inherited a potentially deadly virus from their deceased parents. Therefore, sexual intercourse became highly inappropriate when cross-cousins were socially redefined as siblings.

The mother's sister

As the mother's brother has become less able or less willing to assume the role of guardian, the mother's sister has assumed this responsibility.

According to conceptual models of kinship, the maternal aunt appears to be an ideal guardian. In the levirate, she substituted for her sister. She also assumed pedagogical responsibilities in relation to her nephews and nieces. Several research participants expressed the opinion that the mother's sister's husband was more likely to accept affinally linked orphans into his home than the mother's brother's wife would be. A woman is not linked to her sister's husband by bridewealth and has no authority in his home. Moreover, the children of sisters are classificatory siblings: they are not entitled to special privileges, and sexual intercourse between them is perceived to be incestuous, and therefore unlikely to occur. The prominence of the mother's sister is also an index of the feminisation of childcare, and of her greater chances of being registered as a legal guardian by the welfare bureaucracy than her brother's wife.

Pitso Mashile found her mother's sister and her husband to be far more accommodating to her needs than her mother's brother and his wife. After her mother died in the village, Wendover, her sisters relocated to Impalahoek with their mother. But Pitso remained in Wendover because she was in her final year of high school and could not secure a transfer to a school in Impalahoek. Pitso thus moved to the home of her mother's younger sister.

> My mother's sister [*mangwane*] was kind and asked me to stay with them. If she saw a child she would say, 'This is my child also.' Her husband did not object. He was not working, but said, 'Come and stay here! You are also our child! We will share everything!'

It is significant, however, that most women who acted as guardians of their sister's children were single. Jane Ndlovu, who was a divorcee, said that because she wanted to be in control of her own household, she had no desire to remarry. Thus, she did not feel under any constraint when she decided to accommodate her deceased sister's son. The young man had previously resided with his grandmother, but he experienced profound conflict with his brother. Jane found his presence around the home comforting, because in recent years violent crime had become common in her neighbourhood. Other guardians commended mature girls who provided a helping hand around the home by fetching water, collecting firewood, cooking maize porridge and cleaning.

The mother's sister was more likely than the mother's brother to secure access to foster grants. Nevertheless, the application process was fraught with uncertainties. Denise Monareng filled in 'change of custody' forms for two of her deceased sister's four children who were under the age of 18. After three months, government officials told her that the forms had been 'lost in the system' and asked her to fill in new ones. Another three months later, she received two grants – valued at R310 each. However, according to Denise, the grants were of insufficient value to support the children's needs: she remarked that a single school uniform for one child cost R459. Likewise, Mary Mkhansi and her siblings filled in forms to apply for maintenance and foster grants for their deceased sister's six children. But the outcome was unsuccessful. The social workers told her that the children's biological fathers, who were still alive, were responsible for supporting them financially. Mary said that she had no knowledge of their whereabouts.

Unlike the mother's brother, the mother's sister found it exceptionally difficult to discipline orphaned children – usually a masculine responsibility. Maria Nonyane complained about the behaviour of Albert Mola, the orphaned son of her younger sister. Albert bullied other children in the neighbourhood, dropped out of primary school in 2013, and spent his days at a shopping centre, where he earned tiny amounts of cash by carrying groceries for customers. Maria feared that Albert might become a member of one of the criminal gangs that roamed about the village at night.

The mother's mother

The maternal grandmother (*kokwane*), too, had become a prominent guardian. Grandparents were virtually the last AIDS-free generation, and grandmothers had a deep sense of filial responsibility towards their grandchildren (Block 2014). Under the system of labour migration, elderly women often cared for the children of their married sons, who were working as wage earners in South Africa's industrial centres. They also ended up caring for the children of single, separated and divorced working daughters. However, in the case of parental death, the mother's mother was not seen as a substitute for her surviving daughters; rather, she was a last resort in the absence of any alternative arrangements.

From the viewpoint of orphaned children, the mother's mother was frequently a preferred guardian. Fortes (1949: 236–40) and Radcliffe-Brown (1950) observe that, while interactions between proximate relations in different African contexts are characterised by hierarchy and formality, those between alternate generations often allow for greater equality and even intimacy. This is especially true for maternal grandparents, who are linked to grandchildren as receivers of bridewealth from the marriages of their mothers. This contrast in styles of care is borne out by the experience of Tembisa Ubisi. Tembisa's parents divorced in 1987 when he was merely one year old, and for the next 12 years he lived with his mother and step-father. But his stepfather died in 1999 and his mother in 2002, both from AIDS-related diseases. Tembisa then briefly resided with his father, but soon experienced conflict. 'We had to sleep in the same bed and I wanted to be free. I had a private life and I had girlfriends.' Tembisa also said that his father was often drunk, swore at him, and spread unfounded rumours that he had impregnated several young women. Tembisa eventually chose to live with his maternal grand-mother and found these arrangements to be far more convenient. In her house he had his own room, and, unlike his father, his maternal grandmother tolerated his love affairs.

All grandmothers who were above the age of 60 years had access to state pensions – worth R1,390 per month in 2014 – a valuable form of household income. Pensions had important redistribu-tive effects. In Bushbuckridge, women were more inclined than men to spend their money on resources such as food, and they saw their pensions as a subsidy for the entire household (Schatz and Ogunmefun 2007: 1394). This is linked to the perception that care work is the woman's responsibility, and that it is incumbent on grandmothers to demonstrate love towards their grandchildren in both sentimental and material terms (Weckesser 2011: 40, 91). As legal guardians, grandmothers could also access foster grants on behalf of their grandchildren. Large multi-generational households containing the mother's mother were almost completely dependent on welfare payments.

Bayeforile Mapayile, an 80-year-old woman, was shaken by the successive deaths of her husband, son and two daughters, who all suffered from AIDS-related diseases. In 2014, she lived with her unmarried son, eight grandchildren (including six orphans), and three great-grandchildren. The household relied on Bayeforile's pension, the wages of her son and oldest granddaughter, who both worked as cleaners at a nearby shopping centre, the foster grant for one grandson, and maintenance grants for three great-grandchildren. The household barely made ends meet, and they were obliged to visit the magistrate at three-month intervals so that they could confirm that the family's conditions remained unchanged.

Maternal grandmothers sometimes worked under a great deal of pressure, being burdened with having to care for young dependants in their twilight years, frequently through no choice of their own. The numbers of resident grandchildren in my sample varied from three to nine. Grandmothers were unable to see care as an investment that older children could reciprocate (Weckesser 2011: 95), despite the work that their grandchildren did around the home. Flora Ndlovu, who was 75 years old, cared for five grandchildren (of whom two were orphans) and two great-grandchildren. She told me that, as a mother, she had had to raise her children on her own, and she earned money by selling home-brewed beer to men in the compounds. She had had no opportunity to go to school and did not receive any child maintenance grants. Now, she was still looking after her grand-children, washing them and preparing their lunch boxes before they went to school. This task, she said, was not for the faint-hearted. 'I have no help and I am worn out.' Her older grandchildren caused her stress and depression. 'You can discipline them when they are young, but when they are older they can reply in any way.'

Siblings

Ten of the orphans in sampled households (16 per cent) resided in households that contained no members of older generations. Such households might well be described as 'child-headed' and viewed as an index of desperation, arising from the failure of kinship to provide social care (Sharp and Spiegel 1985). Here, though, the failure of care cannot be generalised to all kinship relations. Where adults proved unreliable, orphans turned to older siblings for assistance. The resilience of this relationship does not merely relate to the struc-tural 'equivalence of siblings' (Radcliffe-Brown 1952a); during the history of labour migration, uterine siblings in rural South Africa often developed mutually supportive bonds, independent of those to their parents (Niehaus 1994).

On some occasions, siblings collectively inherited and managed the homestead of their deceased parents. Prudence Mnisi told me that her parents died in hospital during 2001. At the time, she, a single mother aged 25, was obliged to care for five younger siblings. Prudence's paternal grandparents were resident on a white-owned commercial farm, and only occasionally sent them maize meal. Her paternal aunt, who lived in a nearby village, had been on bad terms with their parents, and their maternal kin were either unable or unpre-pared to help. Prudence secured food parcels from the government for the household, and, with the help of the head teacher of a local school, filled in applications for foster grants for her three younger siblings and maintenance grants for her two sons. (She was awarded these after two years.) Prudence also took up employment at a fruit farm.

Our situation was very pathetic. We sometimes begged
neighbours for food and we went to sleep on empty stomachs.
But it was better when the food parcels came. Every month end
we had to go to Bridgeway – a five-kilometre journey each way –
pushing a wheelbarrow [to fetch the parcels].

But Prudence said that her younger siblings understood their
situation.

Later our father's sister [*rakgadi*] offered to be guardian for one
of the children. But we the children declined the offer. We wanted
to stay together. We did not understand what her aim was. She
might have been after money. It was very important for us to
remain together.

By 2014, three of the Mnisi siblings had married and left home,
and the two sisters remained with Prudence. They were both securely
employed at game lodges. Prudence had clearly distinguished herself
as a most capable guardian.

Conclusions

In South Africa, social scientists, the public and government alike
have displayed broader concern about the effects of HIV/AIDS than
would be predicted by biopolitical theory. Their focus on the status
of survivors has transcended the mere biological status of diseased
individuals. As Bray (2003) shows, analysts of social security systems
expressed great anxiety that the pandemic would provoke crises of
homeless and malnourished orphans, social disorder, and a tidal
wave of criminality. This concern dovetails with the situation in Brazil
and in the Democratic Republic of Congo, where the pandemic has
been linked to a dramatic escalation in the numbers and prominence
of street children (Hecht 1998; De Boeck 2005). In South Africa,
girls and boys have left their rural homes to take up residence in
condemned apartment buildings such as Point Place near Durban's
city centre (Margaretten 2015).

Moreover, the increase in the number of AIDS orphans in places
such as Impalahoek has not brought about a drastic break with the
past, or a discontinuity in institutions responsible for the care and
guardianship of children. Instead, villagers have redeployed older
Northern Sotho and Shangaan kinship models for this purpose.

These models have proven surprisingly resilient, largely due to their flexibility and due to the diffusion of childcare among the parents' siblings and grandparents, and in some cases among the child's own siblings and even their cousins. Far from being a relic of the past, this feature of classificatory kinship structures has proved to be a vital social resource in coping with the harsh effects of the HIV/ AIDS pandemic. Moses Khosa, a middle-aged man whose opinions I greatly value, often spoke about emerging social trends in condemnatory terms. But Moses took immense pride in the fact that there were virtually no orphans resident on the streets of Bushbuckridge.

> It is very hard to find children eating from dustbins at the plaza [shopping] centre. I have only seen one or two of them ... Here it is not like the cities. We have aunts, uncles, *malomes* [mother's brothers] and relatives. If someone dies they take over. We cannot allow children to go orphaned. We are a remote, but civilised area. Here families matter.

Universal definitions of orphan-hood have been elusive, and it has been exceedingly difficult to generalise about the experiences of children whose parents died from AIDS-related diseases. Orphan-hood is a relational construct that denotes a position within networks of consanguinity and affinity. Therefore, the experience of losing a parent is relative to differences in broader kinship structures.

Nonetheless, there are definite limitations to the capacity of kinship to provide appropriate care. As the ethnographic material that I have presented in this chapter shows, children's membership and survival in the reconstituted households have been fraught with social and economic difficulties. The South African social security system – of pensions, child maintenance and foster grants – has also facilitated care. The greater capacity of women relatives of orphans to access social security partially explains the shift from guardianship by paternal to maternal kin, and from guardianship by the mother's brother to the mother's sister. In this context, initiatives such as the Ekuruleni Centre for Orphans and Vulnerable Children provide extremely valuable additional resources that ease the burden of childcare.

8
Conclusions

Nearly three decades have passed since the first cases of HIV/ AIDS were diagnosed in Bushbuckridge. This time period provides the social anthropologist with a unique window through which to perceive some of the complex social patterns and transformations that have become apparent as the devastating pandemic has unfolded. The research I conducted with the aid of Eliazaar Mohlala, and other skilled and experienced local research assistants, occurred under less than perfect conditions, and was limited to a restricted spatial and temporal setting. But many hours of observing diverse social interactions and listening to the voices of different persons affected by sickness in Impalahoek, over month-long periods each year since 1990, have allowed me to rethink some of the central assumptions in current scholarly understandings of HIV/AIDS.

More specifically, the material that I collected has enabled me to appreciate crucial limitations and inadequacies of the 'biopolitical' paradigm, which has become hegemonic in intellectual understandings of HIV and AIDS. The paradigm contends that people across the globe increasingly perceive themselves in somatic terms (Rabinow and Rose 2006), create new forms of sociality (Rose and Novas 2005), and demand resources and rights, based on their membership of biomedical categories (Petryna 2004). In their analysis of the HIV/AIDS pandemic, scholars focus on how the biomedical fraternity has come to exercise 'therapeutic sovereignty' (Nguyen 2010; Decoteau 2013), and on how testing and treatment have ingrained health-based concepts of citizenship (Biehl 2004). Theorists also contend that HIV-infected people use confessional technologies to fashion new selves (Nguyen 2010), and engage in health-based political activism to access antiretroviral medication (Robins 2006).

In Impalahoek, HIV, AIDS-related deaths, biomedical understandings of the pandemic and antiretroviral medication did not arrive *de novo*, on a metaphorical blank slate. They became apparent in a complex ideological field, characterised by well-established and vibrant relational constructs of personhood,[1] metaphysical explanations of misfortune, traditions of divination and healing, and ways of responding to death. The HIV/AIDS pandemic also emerged in a very specific social, political and economic landscape, marked by the establishment of African nationalist rule in the aftermath of apartheid, rapid de-industrialisation, the emergence of a fragile service-based economy, and high dependence on state-provided social security. As rates of marriage declined, older models of kinship, based on consanguinity, have attained special salience.

Biomedical aetiologies of HIV/AIDS did not attain 'instant hegemony' within this complex field of interaction. Nor did their imposition lead to the inevitable dissolution of existing modes of perceiving, treating and dealing with sickness and death. As in many other poorer parts of the world, biomedical facilities were scarce and not nearly as visible as biopolitical theory might suppose (Street 2014). Moreover, during Thabo Mbeki's presidency, the South African government and Health Ministry obstinately refused to 'authorise' biomedical aetiologies of HIV/AIDS and antiretroviral drugs. In 2005, the South African government did launch the large-scale public sector roll-out of HAART. This initiative had the potential to change the course of the pandemic in places such as Impalahoek. Yet, after a decade, only a single HIV clinician, who was also compelled to work in the out-patients department of Tintswalo hospital, was supposed to oversee the distribution of antiretroviral drugs to about 10,000 patients at the Rixile clinic (Versteeg et al. 2013).

Responses at the village level also restricted the hegemony of biomedicine. In this respect, it is significant that interventions to stem the rising tide of HIV infection often took the form of public health education. In clinical practice, unequal relations between doctor and patient are most apparent (Foucault 1973), and in this context patients are most likely to cede power to medical author-ities (Taussig 1980; DiGiacomo 1987). However, as Balshem (1991; 1993) observes, in her study of a cancer prevention project in the city of Philadelphia, public health education is more likely to engender resistance. Health educators claim the power to define issues and assign values to different lifestyles. But the audience does not comprise sick persons in states of vulnerability. She writes: 'The site of community health education is usually a community's home ground ... [here] we can expect to see a community emboldened to speak its mind' (Balshem 1991: 154).

In the village of Impalahoek, biomedical meanings did not displace pre-existing modes of perceiving persons, explaining misfortune, treating the diseased body, constructing sociability and demanding rights. According to Sahlins (1999), 'despondency theory' mistak-enly assumes the inevitable collapse of indigenous cultures, and their degeneration into 'aimless anomie', under the shattering impact of global capitalism. This view, he argues, expresses a loathing of materialism and sentimental pessimism by some in the West (ibid.: 401). Instead, in Impalahoek, the biomedical meanings and modes of treating HIV/AIDS became part of broader, more encompassing ecologies of belief and practice. HIV/AIDS came to be conceptualised, managed and treated not only by physicians and nurses in 'professional' arenas, but also by diviners, Christian healers, fellow church members, kin, neighbours and home-based cares in 'folk' and 'popular' arenas of healthcare (Kleinman 1978). Here, beliefs in pollution, witchcraft, spirit possession, the ancestors and the Holy Spirit were as vital to local understandings and experiences of HIV/AIDS as biomedical constructs of viruses, infections and HAART.

Foucault's (1980) later writings on sexuality provide greater insight into this situation than his earlier studies of medicine and the 'clinical gaze' (Foucault 1973). In Impalahoek, health propagandists, clinicians, nurses and treatment literacy practitioners intervene in the 'vital characteristics of human existence', create discourses, and exercise surveillance over and regulate the bodily conduct of 'citizens'. But their capacity to do so is limited, and these modes of activity are not the only ones worthy of attention. In his studies on sexuality, Foucault (1980) pays far greater attention to the creation of multiple, dispersed and sometimes competing discourses about intimate conduct. These range from religious and psycho-analytic approaches to crude popular ways of speaking about sex. However, as Donham (1998) points out, even in his analysis of sexuality, Foucault does not adequately problematise the role of cultural exchanges across space, and he relies too greatly on medical texts to infer the categories and commitments of ordinary people. Donham's third point of criticism is even more telling. Foucault's notion of discourse, he argues, too frequently assumes the form of a genealogy or unidirectional narrative of supersession. Change, argues Donham, seldom implies the complete replacement of one discourse by another: change tends to be more various, fractured and incomplete. New discourses about sex are more frequently added to older ones and taken up inconsistently and incompletely. This implies a field marked by the simultaneous existence of different, overlapping discourses (ibid.: 11, 15).

It would be erroneous to assume that these divergent discourses and practices exist in any state of coordination or mutual adjustment. While they might well be synchronised (Shaw and Stewart 1994), their coexistence can also assume the forms of confrontation

(Comaroff and Comaroff 2004) or friction (Tsing 2004). The first possibility is apparent in the manner in which, during the initial stages of the pandemic, public health discourses about the incurability of AIDS came together with Christian understandings of leprosy and with vernacular concepts of the 'living dead' and of death as a polluting force. It is the articulation of these discourses, rather than the impositions of biomedicine alone, that explains the stigma of people living with and dying of AIDS. The case of confrontation is more clearly apparent in the relationship between the biomedical diagnosis of AIDS and village-based attributions of witchcraft, which exist in an either/or situation. As we saw in Chapter 3, close kin sometimes denied that their loved ones suffered from AIDS and invoked witchcraft in a bid to deflect blame from existing social and sexual networks. The third – and perhaps most common – relation is one in which diverse orientations exist side by side, without any synthesis or confrontation, in a contingency of incommensurable ontological difference. The parts are serviced independently, with ideas of pollution, spirit possession and witchcraft bearing distinct sources of meaning in times of misfortune (Kiernan 1994). In Chapter 5 we saw how Reggie Ngobeni sequentially deployed different explanatory models to account for his sickness, and how he consulted a variety of healers, who drew on widely different traditions, in his quest for therapy. Reggie constantly tried out and added new concepts, without searching for explanatory consistency. Concepts of pollution, spirit possession and witchcraft often assume the form of 'deep knowledge', existing in hidden, safeguarded spaces, whence formal biomedical orthodoxies can be re-evaluated, subverted and contested (Apter 2007).

It makes greater sense to see the history of HIV/AIDS in Impalahoek in terms of changing configurations of belief and practice, rather than in terms of the linear, progressive diffusion of biopolitics. In the period before the availability of HAART, the stigma of AIDS was most pronounced. This was a product of the way in which public health discourses about the new, inevitably fatal, disease articulated with Christian dogma about sin, and with traditional notions of pollution. During this period, discourses at the village level centred on moral concerns pertinent to the allocation of blame. By invoking conspiracy theories and witchcraft, village residents attempted to counter the tendency towards victim-blaming in biomedical discourses on HIV/AIDS. Conspiracy theories held capricious nurses, racist whites, political agents and corrupt businessmen culpable for the creation and spread of HIV. Accusations of witchcraft, in turn, shifted blame from sexual partners onto envious neighbours and overtly judgemental elders, and changed the focus from intimate sexual networks to strained relations with neighbours and the older generation. Notions about the agency of powerful words, as was evident in the pronouncement that one had tested HIV-positive, enhanced popular anxieties and fears about sickness and death.

The availability of HAART, since 2005, has lessened the stigma of AIDS, has weakened its association with death, and has led to a steady increase in people undertaking tests for HIV antibodies and accessing medication. In this new context, popular discourse gradually drifted away from conspiracies and blame towards treatment and care. But the availability of potentially effective treatment has not diminished the significance of non-biomedical modes of perception and practice. As the life story of Reggie Ngobeni shows, testing for HIV antibodies was frequently a last resort, and HAART was frequently used in combination with other therapies. Reggie's narrative also captures the significance of discreet modes of speaking about HIV and AIDS. Moreover, existing understandings of dreams have formed a template for interpreting, and speaking about, the effects of antiretroviral medication. Another focal concern has been the redeployment of older models of kinship, to provide care for persons suffering from AIDS, and to foster children who have lost parents due to AIDS-related diseases. These arrangements are negotiated in relation to state-provided social security and welfare grants, allocated on the basis of economic vulnerability rather than biological criteria.

My discussions underline the importance of recognising phenomena located well 'beyond the politics of bare life' (Comaroff 2007), and of formulating more appropriate means of understanding, but also of responding to the pandemic.

Culture, South Africa, the baby and the bathwater

There is every danger that new materialist paradigms centred on the body, transnational flows and biological citizenship might well obscure the insights provided by earlier meaning-centred approaches, derived from Kleinman's (1978) attempt to conceptualise medical systems as cultural systems.

Intellectual unease surrounds the very notion of culture. During the 'reflexive turn' of the 1980s and 1990s, anthropologists wrote penetrating critiques of the earlier Boasian approach, which saw culture as the major determinant of consciousness. Boasian scholars treated culture holistically, as geographically specific traits that constituted incommensurate ways of being.[2] Some critics castigated 'ahistorical', 'essentialized', 'simplified', 'reified' and 'rigid' views of culture (Clifford 1998). Others saw traditions as consciously fabricated or 'invented' (Hobsbawm and Ranger 1983) and analysed 'culture talk' as an ideological smokescreen for more fundamental political interests of new elites (Thomas 1992).

Kuper (1994; 2005) is more concerned with subsequent mentalist approaches to culture, as evident in Geertz's (1973) treatment of culture as a system of symbols existing in the minds of social actors. This approach, he argues, incorrectly treats culture as separate and distinct from networks of social relations. For example, Schneider's (1968) analysis of American kinship as a symbolic system takes no cognisance of social class, divorce or regional variations. For Kuper, anthropologists should do more than interpret meaning: we should also elicit conversations between the models of our research subjects and our own theoretical models, and constantly compare social situations. Hence, anthropology should be a cosmopolitan project.

In South Africa, social anthropologists of liberal and left political persuasions have castigated apologists for apartheid who misused an essentialist view of culture to justify racial segregation (Boonzaier and Sharp 1988). This tendency was most pronounced among Afrikaner nationalist anthropologists, called *volkekundiges*, who insisted that the country's population could be divided into distinctive cultural groups, whose purity should be preserved at all costs (Gordon 1988). Critical scholars conducted fieldwork as exposé ethnography, focusing on how systems of political discrimination and economic exploitation rendered people's lives vulnerable, and saw rituals such as beer drinks (McAllister 1991) as forms of resistance to structural marginalisation. In a context in which demonstrations of similarity were crucial to an anti-apartheid position, South African social anthropologists expended much angst in dealing with cultural difference (Gordon and Spiegel 1993: 86).[3]

Nonetheless, different forms of literary criticism have had some impact, as can be seen in attempts by J. Comaroff and J. L. Comaroff (1991: 1997) to study culture as contestable practices, pertinent to historical encounters, such as those between missionaries and Tswana villagers. But new identity struggles in the political domain have engendered new cultural (and even racial) essentialisms. African nationalists condemn the way in which white anthropologists have constructed black subjects as the 'racialised other' and uncritically celebrate a new kind of anthropology at home, or auto-ethnography. They assume that studies by black anthropologists would be radically different in outlook (Nyamnjoh 2012; Boswell 2015).

I agree with many of these critiques. Anthropologists who wish to understand complex, multi-stranded phenomena, such as the South African HIV/AIDS pandemic, cannot remain oblivious to the political uses of culture. Also, any project that reifies culture, or examines symbolic meanings in isolation from broader socio-historical contexts, rests upon mistaken premises. In addition, there is a crucial need for diversity within the community of anthropological scholars, without endorsing essentialism (strategic or otherwise).

But thinking deeply about HIV/AIDS in the light of the ethnographic material that I collected, I am convinced that there is another, equally pertinent, set of dangers associated with casting out the proverbial (cultural) baby with the (essentialist) bathwater. This includes avoiding serious engagement with patterns of meaning, conceptual models, ritual practices and difference – phenomena conventionally discussed under the label of culture. Our anthropological concerns frequently diverge too starkly from those of our research subjects. This is most apparent in the unfashionability of complex phenomena such as kinship, which is vitally important to the way in which villagers construct their moral obligations in everyday social settings (Scheffler 2001). The divergence of concerns is also evident in the manner in which scholars focus on the 'instrumentality' of witchcraft and spirit possession, while paying scant attention to their 'existential' dimensions (Boddy 1994). Such theoretical closures have precluded in-depth interest in the full range of human experience (Van Wyk 2012).

In the light of this discussion, it is essential that we should revise and refine, rather than completely discard, Kleinman's (1978) early attempts to study the cultural dimensions of sickness and healing. Purely materialist analyses are perennially incomplete.

Beyond biomedicine: therapeutic interventions

A nuanced understanding of symbolic meanings, discourses and practices pertinent to lived experiences of sickness, existing in the shadow of biomedicine, has important implications for developing contextually sensitive therapeutic interventions.

An appropriate starting point is Gausset's (2001) critique of reified understandings of culture in the domain of HIV prevention.

Throughout the history of HIV/AIDS in Africa, he argues, social scientists and public health experts alike have treated 'culture' as an obstacle to the attainment of well-being. They have seen exotic practices – ranging from rituals of purification, rites of passage and polygamy to witchcraft beliefs – as contributing towards the rapid spread of HIV.[4] These views externalise culture by seeing it solely as an attribute of 'the other', without recognising the symbolic meanings and social relations inherent in biomedicine. Public health campaigns that fight against unfamiliar, non-biomedical systems of belief can only be counterproductive. For Gausset (ibid.), much is to be gained from configuring the problem not as one of cultural difference (such as dry sex), but rather as one of dangerous cultural practices. Safe sex, he argues, can easily be promoted within the context of both monogamous and polygamous marriages.

Each chapter in this book contributes specific insights for the provision of more effective interventions in the prevention and treatment of HIV/AIDS. Evidence presented in Chapter 2 suggests that, during the earlier phase of the pandemic, the intense stigma of AIDS was partially an outcome of the way in which health education constructed AIDS as a terminal illness. This finding points to the need for critical introspection within the public health fraternity. Evidence also suggests that the creation of hope, which is an important incentive for prevention and treatment, is as much a matter of the cultural redefinition of AIDS as a chronic and serious, yet eminently treatable, condition as it is of simply providing HAART. In this respect, we can learn a great deal from efforts by career patients to destigmatise leprosy. Healthy persons living with AIDS, such as May Mokoena, can do a great deal more to bring the real facts before the public than can fire and brimstone sermons about the need for sexual abstinence during life orientation classes in high schools.

In Chapter 3, I compared the way in which public health discourses, conspiracy theories and witchcraft accusations configure and reconfigure blame for HIV/AIDS. Whereas public health discourses pathologise certain patterns of behaviour among host populations, conspiracy theories construct imaginative links between HIV/AIDS and political and economic relations. These theories largely capture men's anxieties about the capriciousness of a de-industrialising economy. The chapter highlights the need for public health education to incorporate a focus on these broader issues, and to address the gendered concerns of men, who are more likely than women to be alienated from biomedical understandings of HIV and AIDS.

The ethnographic evidence I presented on the power of words warns against the assumption that 'confessional technologies' – such as 'coming out' with HIV positivity – provide a universally appropriate means of confronting the pandemic. These technologies are based on the assumption that speech has the capacity to transform people, combat stigma and bring new hope in contexts of suffering and pain.[5] But it is necessary to recognise differences in the social and cosmological contexts, and in the intrinsic meanings of speech. Unlike urban-based TAC activists, residents of Impalahoek were not able to use 'confessional technologies' to access scarce resources that were associated with the benefits of 'therapeutic citizenship'. In an insecure rural environment, anxiety about the potentially destructive capacity of words – as in cursing, swearing and direct speech about sensitive issues – often outweighed faith in their potential to liberate. The words 'HIV' and 'AIDS' bore negative symbolic loads, and were widely seen to enhance sickness and prophesy death. Many residents avoided or delayed testing for HIV antibodies, out of a fear of being pronounced HIV-positive. In this context, it makes greater sense to treat confession and confidentiality, speech and silence, and direct and euphemistic words as alternative, contextually appropriate modes of dealing with sickness. It is also imperative for health workers to speak with discretion.

In Chapter 5 I presented a critique of the emphasis on 'treatment literacy' in the field of HIV/AIDS prevention and care. Contra the assumptions of health discourses on 'patient responsibility' (Lupton and Petersen 1996), decisions on therapeutic consultations are seldom the product of individual knowledge; more commonly they are made by 'lay therapy management groups'. Also, a constellation of social factors that have little to do with the capacity of individuals to 'interpret information about HIV/AIDS prevention, testing and care' (Schenker 2006: 3) affect the uptake and use of HAART. In a context of radical medical pluralism, in which individuals such as Reggie Ngobeni constantly employ new ways of explaining and treating sickness, without great concern for consistency, treatment literacy may be hard to assess. Non-biomedical explanations of illness that centre on pollution, witchcraft and spirit possession do not necessarily inhibit the effective use of HAART. They may well address non-biological aspects of sickness such as the co-occurrence of different forms of misfortune, anxiety and self-blame. Through indiscriminate opposition to non-biomedical specialists, health programmes may well alienate those they seek to help (Gausset 2001).

In Chapter 6 I elaborated on themes pertaining to social and cultural specificities in the HIV/AIDS pandemic, by showing how the transnational distribution of HAART has not brought a unitary regime of values. I showed how pre-existing frameworks of understanding have shaped the way in which users of HAART interpret vivid and frightening dreams, a biochemical side effect of efavirenz. Research participants saw these dreams as integral to their therapeutic experiences; the dreams attested to the mystical efficacy of antiretroviral drugs. They conferred special insights, battle-hardened dreamers, and constituted a portal through which deceased ancestors and the Holy Spirit provided support. Moreover, by narrating their dream experiences, HAART users communicated anxieties otherwise suppressed in social intercourse. By listening to, rather than dismissing, dream narratives, health workers can access the concerns of HAART users and facilitate better healthcare delivery.

A final set of concerns relate to the care of children who have lost parents to AIDS-related diseases. In Chapter 7 I sought to show how the cosmopolitan concept of 'orphan-hood' does not accurately capture the experiences of such children. I argue that Northern Sotho and Shangaan models of kinship posit a diffusion of parental work, in which the siblings and mothers of the deceased parents, and the siblings of children themselves, become the guardians of their offspring. Hence, the HIV/AIDS pandemic has not generated a crisis of homeless street children in Impalahoek. Additional childcare responsibilities have nonetheless increased the financial hardship of many guardians, who would not have been able to make ends meet without social security payments. Under these conditions, it would make greater sense for social welfare providers to support existing networks of care rather than invest scarce resources in alternative institutions. Social welfare bureaucrats could also recognise the vital obligations of the mother's brother (*malome*) and his wife (*mmamalome*) towards children with deceased parents. Day-care centres for vulnerable children seem more appropriate than full-time orphanages.

Studies focusing on the multi-layered social and cultural dimensions of HIV/AIDS have the capacity to highlight the limitations and mistakes of existing interventions. Most of these problems are not intrinsic to biomedicine itself. In the case of HIV/AIDS, the provision of HAART has drastically improved life expectancies throughout South Africa.[6] Rather, the problems we highlighted seem to be an outcome of one-size-fits-all thinking about the intersection of biomedicine with discourses and practices pertinent to sickness beyond the clinical setting.

Shortly before his unfortunate death due to motor neurone disease, the physician-anthropologist Cecil Helman (2006; 2014) wrote two autobiographical accounts in which he elaborated upon the well-established humanistic critique of techno-scientific medicine, which treats bodies as separate from the unique circumstances of people's lives. Helman defends an older, more holistic style of family practice in which general practitioners, much like shamans, listen sympathetically to patients and help create narratives that make sense of sickness experiences. During the HIV/AIDS pandemic, it was home-based carers who were most attuned to the intersections of different discourses pertinent to the prevention and treatment of people with AIDS in village-based settings. Clinic-based physicians and nurses, church-based Christian healers and diviners possessed more specialised expertise and operated in narrower, more restrictive domains of social intercourse. Home-based carers were accessible, attuned to the social and cultural contexts that mattered, and were a significant presence in the lives of persons living with AIDS. As such, they were uniquely capable of serving as brokers in the delivery of healthcare. However, they were frequently marginalised in health planning and worked as inadequately remunerated volunteers, without any clear vocation (Schneider and Fassin 2002).

Helman (2006; 2014) saw value in subjecting biomedicine to an anthropological gaze. This gaze can highlight limitations and errors – such as the celebration of voyages to Antarctica by a LoveLife campaign in the lowveld. But the more sustained value of medical anthropology is its capacity to bring a perspective to bear on health-related problems that goes beyond the biomedical and beyond biopolitics.

Notes

Preface and acknowledgements

1 I use pseudonyms to describe the fieldwork village and all personal names. This is done to protect the identity of my informants.

2 The speakers of Tsonga are generally known as Shangaan (Mashangane). They are descendants of the subjects of the Zulu chief Soshangane, who came to the South African lowveld, via present day Mozambique, from the late nineteenth century (Niehaus 2002a).

3 Between 1993 and 1999, the number of workers employed in South African gold mining decreased from 428,003 to 195,681; in coal mining from 51,267 to 21,155; in manufacturing from 1,409,977 to 1,286,694; and in construction from 355,114 to 219,797 (SAIRR 2001: 336–8).

4 The early generation of HIV blood tests, which was commonly administered in South Africa, searched the blood sample for antibodies that are created by B-cells in the immune system in response to invasion by HIV. One drawback is that it takes up to 12 weeks for the body to produce enough antibodies to get a positive result. More recent generations of tests search for antigens or for the virus's RNA in the blood sample. These tests are sensitive within a window of only two weeks.

Chapter 1

1 See Niehaus et al. (2001: 228–35) for an earlier and more in-depth discussion of my fieldwork methods.

2 According to Rabinow and Rose (2006) contemporary 'biological citizenship' differs from that prevailing in the eighteenth century, when states sought to preserve the nation as a biological entity, as seen in terms of bloodlines and in-built moral capacities. States no longer entertain unitary concepts of the nation, nor simplistic notions of race and eugenics, but they still concern themselves with the biological essence of citizenry. Moreover, states disseminate scientific information to shape the interpretive gaze of citizens.

3 Nguyen (2010) claims that this situation finds a historical precedent in the discriminatory allocation of biomedical resources in colonial times, exacerbating distinctions between Europeans, African middle classes, and the population at large.

4 These transcriptase inhibitors, even when administered only in the latter stages of pregnancy, significantly reduced chances of mother–child transmission of HIV. The South African Health Department argued that these drugs attacked inoffensive microbes and did not combine well with tuberculosis medication.

5 During 2006, only 141,346 of an envisaged 456,650 South African public-sector patients were receiving treatment (Natrass 2006: 620).

6 Meinert (2014: 119) also observes the importance of 'homework' – instructions on eating, taking medication and practising safe sex – in antiretroviral treatment (ART) programmes. Such work is carried out in domestic contexts and deeply ingrained in sociality centred on kinship.

7 Apart from pockets of activism such as those associated with

the urban-based TAC, HAART programmes usually steer clear of transformative politics (Marsland and Prince 2012). HIV-positive persons are generally more concerned with accessing resources than with agitating for rights in relation to the state (Prince 2013: 30).

8 Reclamation and Resettlement Report, Native Affairs Department, Bushbuckridge 1957, NTS 17/423/1, V10226, Government Archives, Hamilton Street, Pretoria.

9 *Nzunzu* was believed to capture people and submerge them in deep rivers. They did not drown, but lived underwater, breathing like fish. Only after their kin had slaughtered a cow for *nzunzu* would it release its captives. They crawled from the water on their knees and emerged as powerful diviners with a wide assortment of herbs. This myth resonates with the experience of birth. The foetus, too, lives in fluids, inside the womb (Hirst 1993).

10 During the mid-1990s, there were 27 churches in Impalahoek, with a combined total membership of 6,000 adult baptised members: 75 per cent of Christians belonged to 'Zionist-type' churches; 16 per cent to 'Pentecostal-type'; and only 9 per cent to missionary churches such as the Methodists (Niehaus et al. 2001: 31–6).

11 Under the terms of the Act, anyone who indicated that another person was a witch or approached 'witch doctors' to 'sniff out' witches could be fined up to R2,000 (about £130), or imprisoned for up to ten years. Should the person accused of witchcraft be killed, the perpetrators could be jailed for up to 20 years.

12 Bushbuckridge was initially allocated to Limpopo Province, but residents soon complained about inadequate service delivery

and demanded that the region be incorporated into Mpumalanga Province instead. They formed a Border Crisis Committee, which launched a 'rolling mass action', comprising protest marches, strikes and boycotts, in support of its demands. But only in 2005 did government transfer Bushbuckridge to Mpumalanga.

13 See Ferguson (2015) for an extensive discussion of South Africa's social welfare system. He argues that social protectionism became a key domain of policy innovation, in response to post-apartheid political expectations. In South Africa, pensions and other grants were paid to more than 16 million persons (some 30 per cent of the country's population). The grants reached some 44 per cent of households nationwide (ibid.: 6).

14 Agincourt is located 20 kilometres south of Impalahoek. During 2000, the Agincourt study population comprised 68,631 persons residing in 11,212 households in 21 village sections.

15 A CD4 count refers to the number of CD4 T lymphocytes in a blood sample. These are a type of white blood cell that activate the body's immune system but are destroyed by HIV. In HIV-positive people, the CD4 count is the most important laboratory indicator of how well their immune system is working and is the strongest predictor of HIV progression. Adults who are in good health generally register a CD4 count of from 500 to 1,200 cells/mm^3.

16 By that time, 25 per cent of all women receiving antenatal care and 64 per cent of patients undergoing HIV tests at Tintswalo hospital were confirmed as seropositive (MacPherson et al. 2008: 589).

17 Between 2011 and 2013, six medical specialists resigned from Tintswalo. These included

specialists in orthopaedics, anaesthesia, emergency services, surgery and paediatrics (Versteeg et al. 2013).

Chapter 2

1 Mbali (2004) interprets the government's AIDS denial as a reaction to the colonial construction of Africans as having inherently diseased sexuality. She concurs with Stoler's (1995) argument that European nations were differentiated from sexualised 'others' in the colonies.

2 The relative absence of stigma that adheres to masculine promiscuity is dramatically illustrated by public reactions during the rape trail of Jacob Zuma, South Africa's former deputy president. Zuma readily admitted to having engaged in unprotected extramarital sex with an HIV-positive woman half his age. This happened while his daughter slept in the same home. Yet, according to one survey, 55 per cent of black respondents wanted Zuma to become South Africa's next president. In a show of support, Senzeni Zokwana, president of the National Union of Mineworkers, said that his union 'did not adhere to the Ten Commandments and did not need Christians to tell it that adultery was wrong' (Monare 2006).

3 In citing these comments, I do not endorse the view that deadly routine infections such as tuberculosis are separable from AIDS. In the Agincourt district of Bushbuckridge, tuberculosis accounted for 26 per cent of the immediate causes of AIDS deaths (Zwang et al. 2007).

4 Throughout colonial Africa, Christian mission societies took responsibility for the treatment of lepers and projected powerful disease symbols onto Africa. Leper settlements were places of isolation in which the Christian message was presented as the only sign of hope (Vaughan 1991: 77–99). Also, see Silla's (1998) analysis of how leprosy sufferers became social outcasts in Mali and Deacon's (2003) work on the historical use of Robben Island as a leprosarium.

5 E. J. Krige and J. Krige (1965 [1943]) write that, in the northern parts of the lowveld, rulers 'were not allowed to become old or decrepit, lest their kingdom suffer; and either they committed suicide, or they were killed'. They observe that, among the Lobedu, 'tradition decrees that the queen shall have no physical defect and must poison herself' if she becomes ill.

6 Villagers believed that, like one's conscience, the *thefifi* of a murdered person could haunt a murderer and force him to confess. This condition closely resembled the well-known case of *nueer* among the Nuer of Southern Sudan, where the murderer had a mystical bond with the victim and was so polluted that only a leopard-skin priest could cure him through blood-letting (Hutchinson 1998).

7 In a study of 298 tuberculosis patients at the Tintswalo hospital, Pronyk (2001) determined a median delay of ten weeks between the onset of symptoms and the initiation of hospital treatment. In 14 cases the total delay exceeded one year. Many patients first sought help from spiritual and traditional healers (ibid.: 264).

8 Deacon (2002) does explore local interpretation to some extent.

Chapter 3

1 Sobo (1993) highlights the importance of sustaining 'wisdom' and monogamy' narratives for the maintenance of self-respect and esteem among inner-city African American women. Women take pride in their ability to judge men and identify 'clean' (disease-free)

and 'conscious' (upstanding) men, and in their ability to sustain long-term sexual relationships. These narratives are also apparent in Bushbuckridge.

2 Sanders and West (2003) define conspiracy theories as attempts to attribute unexplained events to a sinister plot. They argue for certain similarities between conspiracy theories and occult cosmologies, most notably in the belief that powers work in unpredictable and capricious ways within realms normally concealed from view. However, conspiracy theories concern themselves with a smaller part of the world's workings (ibid.: 7).

3 See Andersson (2002), Ashforth (2002), Probst (1999), Schoepf (1988; 2001) and Yamba (1997).

4 See J. Comaroff and J. L. Comaroff (1987) and James (1999) for more extensive discussions of the rhetorical uses of *setšo* and *sekgowa* in South Africa. Van der Vliet (1991) explores the gendered dimension of this contrast, particularly as it pertains to marriage.

5 These perceptions correspond to the different attitudes of women and men concerning the introduction of female condoms in South Africa and in Kenya. Kaler (2001) reports that women saw female condoms as facilitating their autonomy, self-determination and empowerment. Men, however, regarded female condoms as a dangerous threat to masculinity. Rumours circulated among men that the condoms might be laced with HIV, get lost inside the woman, or be used by women to collect sperm for bewitching men (ibid.: 793).

6 Leclerc-Madlala (1997; 2002) records claims that young Zulu men who are HIV-positive deliberately spread the virus so that they need not die alone, and they believe that they can be cured by having sex with a virgin. In

these matters, it is hard to separate fact from fiction, and these claims may well be no more than myths about myths. I have not recorded any beliefs in the virgin cleansing myth in Bushbuckridge.

7 On AIDS and conspiracy theories, see Farmer (1992: 230–43), Hellinger (2003), Schoepf (2001: 341–2) and Treichler (1999: 220–6).

8 Before the South African elections of 1994, ANC activists warned villagers that the members of right-wing political formations had delivered poisoned bread to local schools and dumped poisoned milk next to village roads. They also alleged that white farmers distributed potatoes stained with invisible election ink at local markets and churches. When the hands of those who touched the potatoes were scanned under ultraviolet light at the polling stations, it would indicate that they had already voted (Niehaus et al. 2001: 76–81).

9 See Niehaus (2000b) for a discussion of medicine murders in Bushbuckridge. White (2000) and Murray and Sanders (2005) provide more extensive analysis of such beliefs and practices in the cases of Central Africa and Lesotho in colonial times.

Chapter 4

1 See Nguyen (2009; 2010) for a detailed genealogy of confessional technologies. He argues that these technologies depend on the following assumptions: people can take control of their own lives by working on themselves; the ability to heal requires that one first overcomes personal sickness; secrets untold become pathogens; and the experience of sharing secrets is cathartic and healing.

2 A similar trend is apparent in neighbouring Botswana. During 2001, the government of

Botswana launched an extremely comprehensive programme of free testing and treatment. After two years, only 15,000 people had come forward to utilise these facilities (Steinberg 2008: 1). However, by 2005, government had administered about 158,000 tests (Klaits 2010: 39).

3 South Africans who test HIV-positive and register a CD4 count of 200 in 2005 (currently 250) or less are judged incapable of working and are entitled to receive monthly disability grants; these were valued at R780 (approximately £50) in 2005. The grants frequently constituted a significant source of income in poor households (Leclerc-Madlala 2006).

4 In a study of 25 men who received HAART at Rixile clinic, Mfecane (2011: 133) found that only one of his research participants had tested for HIV antibodies before becoming severely ill. Most men tried hard to disguise their symptoms of AIDS.

5 Danger is generally more apparent when words are spoken in the mother tongue. However, the words 'HIV' and 'AIDS' seemed to have special power because they had recently become part of the vernacular. People were being forced to bring words into their language they saw as bringing misfortune into society.

6 See McAllister's (2006) discussion of the significance of oratory in beer drinks, which are held to welcome home migrant labourers and thank the ancestors for having protected them during their sojourn, in Xhosa-speaking households in the Eastern Cape.

7 See de Heusch's (1980) analysis of the analogy between birth and the baking and firing of clay pots among Tsonga-speaking people.

8 A belief in the malevolent power of words is evident in the case of persons called *sahir* in Northern Sudan, where people attribute the casting of evil to utterances in the form of metaphors, rather than gazes (Ibrahim 1994).

9 Residents of Bushbuckridge conceptualised termites – along with snakes and moles – as creatures from below, and associated them with dead humans, who lie buried beneath the soil. For this reason, they frequently saw termite hills as portals, connecting the realms of the living and the dead. People sometimes poured libations of beer for the ancestors on termite hills and saw the anomalous appearance of a termite hill in one's yard as an omen of death. Diviners sometimes buried the mucus of epileptics in termite hills to destroy their sickness.

Chapter 5

1 Epidemiological surveys have noted that, even under optimal conditions of supply, the uptake of ARVs and adherence to therapy in South Africa vary widely between different locations and have been less than satisfactory (see George 2006; Gill et al. 2005; Dahab et al. 2011).

2 Graham et al. (2007) found that 64 per cent of patients with at least ninth-grade reading skill levels took 95 per cent of their ARV medication, as indexed by pharmacy refills, compared with only 40 per cent of patients with lower reading skill levels.

3 See Ashforth's (2010) discussions of the pitfalls of translation work in internationally funded programmes.

4 In 2004, South Africans were eligible for ARVs only if they registered a CD4 count of 200 or less. The threshold increased to 350 in 2009 and again to 500 January 2015. As from September 2016, all South Africans who test positive for HIV are eligible for

ARVs, irrespective of their CD4 counts.

5 The Ndzau spirits allegedly came from Musapa in Mozambique and possessed the descendants of the Shangaan soldiers who killed them in the battles of the mid-nineteenth century (see Honwana 2003). These spirits were known to be particularly powerful.

6 In the South African demographic landscape, the term 'coloured' denotes a broad and heterogeneous population category. It refers to people considered to be descendants of the indigenous Khoisan population, as well as people descended from mixed-race couples.

7 Reggie's experiences concur with research findings that show hunger to be a principal complaint of people on ARV treatment (Kalofonos 2010).

8 See Kleinman's (1995: 1–20) auto-critique of his earlier writings, in particular his account of the limitations of his earlier concept of 'explanatory paradigms' in the field of medical anthropology.

Chapter 6

1 For more recent anthropological studies on the circulation of pharmaceuticals, see Petryna et al. (2006), Biehl (2006; 2007), Dumit (2012) and Peterson (2014).

2 Berglund observed that many Zulu diviners place the plant *imphepho* under their pillows so that their dreams might be clear. This, they told him, is because 'dreams are the most important thing to us' (Berglund 1976: 114).

3 In Bushbuckridge, tuberculosis was the single most common cause of death among HIV-positive persons (MacPherson et al. 2008: 588).

4 In the South African lowveld, people are said to 'drink' (*enwa* in Northern Sotho) tablets, whereas in Standard English people 'take' tablets.

5 The descriptions of Mfecane (2011), who had conducted extensive participant observation at the same clinic, match their accounts about these instructions.

6 Nearly all ARVs cause nausea, vomiting and diarrhoea. Other specific reactions are mitochondrial toxicity; hypersensitivity, including rashes, fever, fatigue and mucosal ulceration; lipodystrophy syndrome; anaemia; poor concentration; alopecia; bone marrow suppression; dizziness; impaired concentration; and hepatitis. Besides vivid dreams, which occur in the first few days or weeks, patients using efavirenz might also experience mania and impaired concentration. These side effects usually resolve spontaneously (Carr and Cooper 2000).

7 Also see Dahab et al. (2011).

8 During the Marikana massacre, which took place in August 2012, members of the South African police service shot and killed 41 striking workers at the Lonmin platinum mine. Although the shootings happened close to Rustenburg, images of them were repeatedly screened on television, and they were widely discussed in Impalahoek.

9 The theme of receiving money was the focus of three ARV-induced dreams (see the dreams of Reggie Ngobeni and Jane Nyalungu). Any interpretation of these dreams as connoting wish fulfilment seems over simplistic. The appearance of money in non-ARV-induced dreams might well be seen to be an omen of death. This interpretation is informed by the collection of cash at funerals, and is based on the perception that precious metals, from which coins are made, come from beneath the soil, which is the domain of the dead.

Diviners generally treat money as 'hot', and they cool coins or notes they receive by rubbing them in ash. Due to its uncontrolled circulation, money bears the substances of unknown persons and may therefore be an agent of pollution or an instrument of witchcraft (Comaroff 1985: 187).

10 The mystical powers of ARVs were apparent in their non-medical use. During fieldwork, I constantly heard rumours that young thieves, who were known to engage in crimes such as housebreaking and theft, stole the ARVs of patients walking home from Rixile clinic. The rascals then crushed the ARVs, mixed their powder with cannabis, and manufactured a concoction called *nyaope* (*hunga*; literally 'river fish' in Tsonga). When smoked, *nyaope* allegedly had potent hallucinatory effects that released users from their daily concerns and bestowed on them feelings of confidence and immense bravery. I was unable to interview anyone who had smoked ARVs.

Chapter 7

1 *Sarafina!* is a well-known South African musical about the 1976 uprisings.

2 See Manona (1980), Murray (1981), Spiegel (1986), Niehaus (1988) and Townsend (1997).

3 They use the concept of 'households' to refer to co-resident individuals who 'eat from the same pot' and 'kinship' to denote broader relations of affinity and consanguinity (Ansell and van Blerk 2004: 676).

4 In terms of specialist kinship jargon, the Northern Sotho model of kinship is classically 'Iroquois' and the Shangaan one a variant of the 'Omaha' type (see Lane and Lane 1959).

5 The corresponding Tsonga terms are *tatana* (father), *bavankulu* (father's older brother),

bavantsongo (father's younger brother), *hahani* (father's sister), *manana* (mother), *mhaninkulu* (mother's older sister), *mhanintsonga* (mother's younger sister) and *malume* (mother's brother).

6 MZ – mother's sister; FB – father's brother. Other abbreviations used in the text are: MB – mother's brother; FZ – father's sister; MBd – mother's brother's daughter; MBs – mother's brother's son; FZd – father's sister's daughter; and FZs – father's sister's son.

7 The discrepancy in the figures of married men and women is explained by the presence of polygyny in a few exceptional cases.

8 Two male and ten female research participants were not married and did not have sexual partners during the time of sickness.

9 The term *mohlokomedi* denotes someone who temporarily borrows cattle from a wealthy stock owner under the *mafisa* system, takes care of them, and benefits from their produce.

Chapter 8

1 Relational modalities of personhood imply that the person is not defined purely in terms of internal qualities and seen as self-enclosed. Instead, there is an emphasis on how the person is defined through relations, and involved in processes of being added to, and built upon, by others (LiPuma 1998). The latter is apparent in Bushbuckridge, where the person is an amalgam of flesh (*mmele*), blood (*madi*), breath (*moya*) and aura (*seriti*) (Niehaus 2002b).

2 The earlier, more holistic view is perhaps most clearly articulated in Kroeber's (1917) exceedingly broad formulation of culture as the 'super-organic'.

3 Such angst was already apparent in Gluckman's (1975) venomous

attack on Leach's structural approach, in which he argued that Leach's notion of translating unique cultures led to a position close to that of the adherents of apartheid. In retrospect, Gluckman's attack seems misplaced, based on an inadequate grasp of the universalistic implications implicit in Leach's structural approach of symbols, and unappreciative of Leach's anti-authoritarian and humanist political position.

4 One notable exception relates to the promotion of male circumcision, an indigenous cultural practice that is believed to render some protection against HIV infection, by public health campaigns (Halperin and Bailey 1999).

5 These assumptions about words accord with classical anthropological observations that the potency of ritual lies as much in the uttering of words as in the manipulation of objects (Malinowski 1966; Tambiah 1968; Lévi-Strauss 1963).

6 The South African Medical Research Council (2015) estimates that life expectancy in South Africa showed a staggering increase of 8.5 years between 2005 and 2013.

References

Agamben, G. (1998) *Homo Sacer: sovereign power and bare life.* Stanford CA: Stanford University Press.

— (2005) *States of Exception.* Chicago IL: University of Chicago Press.

Andersson, J. (2002) 'Sorcery in the era of "Henry IV": kinship, mobility and morality in Buhera District, Zimbabwe', *Journal of the Royal Anthropological Institute* 8 (3): 425–99.

Ansell, N. and L. van Blerk (2004) 'Children's migration as a household/family strategy: coping with AIDS in Lesotho and Malawi', *Journal of Southern African Studies* 30 (3): 673–90.

Appadurai, A. (1986) 'Introduction' in A. Appadurai (ed.), *The Social Life of Things: commodities in cultural perspective.* Cambridge: Cambridge University Press.

— (1996) *Modernity at Large: cultural dimensions of globalization.* Minneapolis MN: University of Minnesota Press.

Apter, A. (2007) *Beyond Words: discourse and cultural agency in Africa.* Chicago IL: University of Chicago Press.

Ashforth, A. (2002) 'An epidemic of witchcraft? Implications of AIDS for the post-apartheid state', *African Studies* 61 (1): 121–44.

— (2005) *Witchcraft, Violence and Democracy in South Africa.* Chicago IL: University of Chicago Press.

— (2010) 'Spiritual insecurity and AIDS in South Africa' in H. Dilger and U. Luig (eds), *Morality, Hope and Grief: anthropologies of AIDS in Africa.* Oxford: Berghahn Books.

Ashforth, A. and N. Natrass (2005) 'Ambiguities of "culture" and the antiretroviral rollout in South Africa', *Social Dynamics* 31 (2): 285–303.

Bahre, E. (2007) 'Reluctant solidarity: death, urban poverty and neighbourly assistance in South Africa', *Ethnography* 8 (1): 33–59.

Balshem, M. (1991) 'Cancer, control and causality: talking about cancer in a working-class community', *American Ethnologist* 18 (1): 152–72.

— (1993) *Cancer in the Community: class and medical authority.* Washington DC: Smithsonian Institution Press.

Bangsberg, D., S. Perry, E. Charlebois, R. Clark, M. Robertson, A. Zolopa and A. Moss (2001) 'Non-adherence to highly active antiretroviral therapy predicts progression to AIDS', *AIDS* 15 (9): 1181–3.

Bank, A. and L. Bank (eds) (2013) *Inside African Anthropology: Monica Wilson and her interpreters.* New York NY: Cambridge University Press.

Basso, K. (1969) *Western Apache Witchcraft.* Tucson AZ: University of Arizona Press.

Berglund, A.-I. (1976) *Zulu Thought-Patterns and Symbolism.* Uppsala: Swedish Institute of Mission Research.

Bhat, V., M. Ramburuth, M. Singh, O. Titi, A. Antony, L. Chiya and E. Irusen (2010) 'Factors associated with poor adherence to anti-retroviral therapy in patients attending a rural health center in South Africa', *European Journal of Clinical Microbiology and Infectious Diseases* 29 (8): 947–53.

Biehl, J. (2004) 'The activist state: global pharmaceuticals, AIDS and citizenship in Brazil', *Social Text* 22 (3): 105–32.

— (2006) 'Will to live: AIDS drugs and local economies of salvation',

Public Culture 18 (3): 457–72.
— (2007) *Will to Live: AIDS therapies and the politics of survival*. Princeton NJ: Princeton University Press.

Bloch, M. (1988) 'Death and the concept of a person' in C. Cederroth, C. Corlin and J. Lundstrom (eds), *On the Meanings of Death: essays on mortuary rituals and eschatological beliefs*. Stockholm, Almqvist and Wicksell International.

Block, E. (2014) 'Flexible kinship: caring for AIDS orphans in rural Lesotho', *Journal of the Royal Anthropological Institute* 20 (4): 711–27.

Boddy, J. (1994) 'Spirit possession revisited: beyond instrumentality', *Annual Review of Anthropology* 23: 407–34.

Boonzaier, E. and J. Sharp (eds) (1988) *South African Keywords: the uses and abuses of political concepts*. Cape Town: David Philip.

Bornstein, E. (2001) 'Child sponsorship, evangelism, and belonging in the work of World Vision Zimbabwe', *American Ethnologist* 28 (3): 595–622.

Boswell, R. (2015) 'Anthropology in Southern Africa: an-other perspective', *American Anthropologist* 117 (4): 761–2.

Bourdieu, P. (1991) *Language and Symbolic Power*. Cambridge MA: Harvard University Press.

Boyce, P. (2007) 'Conceiving kothis: men who have sex with men in India and the cultural subject of HIV prevention', *Medical Anthropology* 26 (2): 175–203.

Bray, R. (2003) 'Predicting social consequences of orphanhood in South Africa', *African Journal of AIDS Research* 2 (1): 39–55.

Butt, L. (2005) '"Lipstick girls" and "fallen women": AIDS and conspiratorial thinking in Papua, Indonesia', *Cultural Anthropology* 20 (3): 412–42.
— (2011) 'Can you keep a secret? Pretenses of confidentiality

in HIV/AIDS counseling and treatment in eastern Indonesia', *Medical Anthropology* 30 (3): 319–38.

Butt, L and R. Eves (eds) (2008) *Making Sense of AIDS: culture, sexuality and power in Melanesia*. Honolulu HI: University of Hawai'i Press.

Carr, A. and D. Cooper (2000) 'Adverse effects of antiretroviral therapy', *Lancet* 356: 1423–30.

Chandler, D. L. (2013) 'Dr Death found guilty of creating drugs, chemicals to kill Africans', Newsone, 20 December. Available at: https://newsone.com/2814931/doctor-death-south-africa-wouter-basson-guilty (accessed 7 July 2018).

Ciekawy, D. and P. Geschiere (1998) 'Containing witchcraft: conflicting scenarios in postcolonial Africa', *African Studies Review* 41 (3): 1–14.

Clifford, J. (1998) *The Predicament of Culture: twentieth century ethnography, literature and art*. Cambridge MA: Harvard University Press.

Collins, T. and J. Stadler (2000) 'Love, passion and play: sexual meanings amongst youth in the Northern Province of South Africa', *Journal des Anthropologues* 82 (83): 325–38.

Comaroff, J. (1985) *Body of Power, Spirit of Resistance: the culture and history of a South African people*. Chicago IL: University of Chicago Press.
— (2007) 'Beyond bare life: AIDS (bio)politics and the neoliberal order', *Public Culture* 19 (1): 197–220.

Comaroff, J. and J. L. Comaroff (1987) 'The madman and the migrant: work and labour in the historical consciousness of a South African people', *American Ethnologist* 14 (2): 191–209.
— (1991) *Of Revelation and Revolution. Volume 1: Christianity, colonialism and consciousness in South Africa*. Chicago IL:

University of Chicago Press.
— (1997) *Of Revelation and Revolution. Volume 2: The dialectics of modernity on a South African frontier*. Chicago IL: University of Chicago Press.
— (2004) 'Criminal justice, cultural justice: the limits of liberalism and the pragmatics of difference in the new South Africa', *American Ethnologist* 31 (2): 188–204.

Cooper, F. (2001) 'What is the concept of globalization good for? An African historian's perspective', *Africa Affairs* 100 (399): 189–213.

Curley, R. (1983) 'Dreams of power: social process in a West African religious movement', *Africa* 53 (3): 20–38.

Dahab, M., K. Kielmann, S. Charalambous, A. Karstaedt, R. Hamilton, L. La Grange, K. Fielding, G. Churchyard and A. Grant (2011) 'Discontinuation of therapy often too high: contrasting reasons for discontinuation of antiretroviral therapy in workplace and public-sector HIV programs in South Africa', *AIDS Patient Care and STDS* 25 (1): 53–9.

Deacon, H. (2002) *Understanding AIDS Stigma: a theoretical and methodological analysis*. Cape Town: Human Sciences Research Council Press.
— (2003) 'Patterns of exclusion on Robben Island, 1654–1992' in C. Strange and A. Bashforth (eds), *Isolation: places and practices of exclusion*. London: Routledge.

De Beer, C. (1984) *Health and Health Care in Mhala: an overview*. Carnegie Conference Paper. Cape Town: Southern Africa Labour and Development Research Unit (SALDRU), University of Cape Town.

De Boeck, F. (2005) 'The divine seed: children, gift and witchcraft in the Democratic Republic of Congo' in A. Honwana and F. De Boeck (eds), *Makers and Breakers: children and youth in postcolonial Africa*. Oxford: Currey.

Decoteau, C. (2013) *Ancestors and Antiretrovirals: the biopolitics of HIV/AIDS in postapartheid South Africa*. Chicago IL: University of Chicago Press.

de Heusch, L. (1980) 'Heat, physiology, and cosmogony: rites de passage among the Thonga' in I. Karp and C. S. Bird (eds), *Explorations in African Systems of Thought*. Bloomington IN: Indiana University Press.

Delius, P. and C. Glaser (2005) 'Sex, disease and stigma in South Africa: historical perspectives', *African Journal of AIDS Research* 4 (1): 29–36.

De Waal, M. (2013) 'A case of sick clinical management at Mpumalanga's Tintswalo hospital', *Daily Maverick*, 14 March. Available at: www.dailymaverick.co.za/article/2013-03-14-a-case-of-sick-clinical-management-at-mpumalangas-tintswalo-hospital/#.V8FmAo9OJMs (accessed 27 August 2016).

DiGiacomo, S. (1987) 'Biomedicine as a cultural system: an anthropologist in the kingdom of the sick' in H. Baer (ed.), *Encounters with Biomedicine*. New York NY: Gordon and Breach.

Dilger, H. and U. Luig (eds) (2010) *Morality, Hope and Grief: anthropologies of AIDS in Africa*. Oxford: Berghahn Books.

Dold, T. and M. Cocks (2000) 'The *iNtelezi* plants of the Eastern Cape: traditional and contemporary medicines', *Aloe* 37 (1): 10–13.

Donham, D. (1998) 'Freeing South Africa: the modernization of male–male sexuality in Soweto', *Cultural Anthropology* 13 (1): 3–21.

Douglas, M. (1970) *Purity and Danger*. Harmondsworth: Penguin.

Dumit, J. (2012) *Drugs for Life: how pharmaceutical companies define our health*. Durham NC: Duke University Press.

Durham, D. and F. Klaits (2002) 'Funerals and the public space of sentiment in Botswana', *Journal of Southern African Studies* 28 (4): 777–95.

Etkin, N. (1991) 'Cultural constructions of efficacy' in S. van der Geest and S. Reynolds Whyte (eds), *The Contexts of Medicines in Developing Countries: studies in pharmaceutical anthropology.* Amsterdam: Het Spinhuis.

— (1992) 'Side-effects: cultural constructions and reinterpretations of Western pharmaceuticals', *Medical Anthropology Quarterly* 6 (1): 99–113.

Evans-Pritchard, E. (1937) *Witchcraft, Oracles and Magic among the Azande.* Oxford: Clarendon Press.

Eves, R. (2012) 'Resisting global AIDS knowledges: born-again Christian narratives of the epidemic from Papua New Guinea', *Medical Anthropology* 31 (1): 61–76.

Farmer, P. (1992) *Aids and Accusation: Haiti and the geography of blame.* Berkeley CA: University of California Press.

Fassin, D. (2007) *When Bodies Remember: experiences and politics of AIDS in South Africa.* Berkeley CA: University of California Press.

Fassin, D., F. le Marcis and T. Lethata (2008) 'Life and times of Magda A: telling a story of violence in South Africa', *Current Anthropology* 49 (2): 225–347.

Feierman, S. (1990) *Peasant Intellectuals: anthropology and history in Tanzania.* Madison WI: University of Wisconsin Press.

Ferguson, J. (1990). *The Anti-politics Machine: 'development' and bureaucratic power in Lesotho.* Cambridge: Cambridge University Press.

— (1999) *Expectations of Modernity: myths and meanings of urban life on the Zambian Copperbelt.* Berkeley CA: University of California Press.

— (2006) 'Decomposing modernity: history and hierarchy after development' in *Global Shadows: Africa in the neoliberal world order.* Durham NC: Duke University Press.

— (2015) *Give a Man a Fish: reflections on the new politics of distribution.* Durham NC: Duke University Press.

Fordham, G. (2004) *A New Look at Thai AIDS: perspectives from the margin.* New York NY and Oxford: Berghahn Books.

Fortes, M. (1949) *The Web of Kinship among the Tallensi.* Oxford: Oxford University Press.

Foucault, M. (1973) *The Birth of the Clinic.* New York NY: Pantheon Books.

— (1977) *Discipline and Punish: the birth of the prison.* London: Penguin.

— (1980) *The History of Sexuality: Volume 1.* New York NY: Vintage.

Freeman, C. (2001) 'Is local: global as feminine: masculine? Rethinking the gender of globalisation', *Signs* 26 (4): 1007–36.

Freud, S. (1994 [1900]) *The Interpretation of Dreams.* New York NY: Barnes and Noble.

Gallant, M. and E. Maticka-Tyndale (2004) 'School-based HIV prevention programmes for African youth', *Social Science and Medicine* 58: 1337–51.

Galt, A. (1982) 'The evil eye as synthetic image and its meanings on the island of Pantelleria, Italy', *American Ethnologist* 9 (4): 664–81.

Garner, R. (2000) 'Safe sects? Dynamic religion and AIDS in South Africa', *Journal of Modern African Studies* 38 (1): 41–69.

Gausset, Q. (2001) 'AIDS and cultural practices in Africa: the case of the Tonga (Zambia)', *Social Science and Medicine* 52: 509–18.

Geertz, C. (1973) *The Interpretation of Cultures: selected essays.* New York NY: Basic Books.

Geffin, N. (2005) 'Echoes of Lysenko: state-sponsored pseudo-science in South Africa', *Social Dynamics* 31 (2): 183–210.

Geissler, P. and F. Becker (eds) (2009) *AIDS and Religious Practice in Africa*. Leiden: Brill.

Geissler, P. and R. Prince (2012) *The Land is Dying: contingency, creativity and conflict in Western Kenya*. Oxford: Berghahn Books.

George, G. (2006) 'Workplace ART programs: why do companies invest in them and are they working?', *African Journal of AIDS Research* 5 (2): 179–88.

Germond, P. and J. Cochrane (2010) 'Health worlds: conceptualizing landscapes of health and healing', *Sociology* 44 (2): 307–24.

Geschiere, P. (1998) 'Globalization and the power of indeterminate meaning: witchcraft and spirit cults in Africa and East Asia', *Development and Change* 29: 811–37.

Gevisser, M. (2007) *Thabo Mbeki: the dream deferred*. Cape Town: Jonathan Ball.

Gill, C., D. Hamer, J. Simon, D. Thea and L. Sabin (2005) 'No room for complacency about adherence to antiretroviral therapy in sub-Saharan Africa', *AIDS* 19 (12): 1243–9.

Gluckman, M. (1975) 'Anthropology and apartheid: the work of South African anthropologists' in M. Fortes and M. Patterson (eds), *Studies in African Social Anthropology*. London: Academic Press.

Goffman, E. (1971) *Stigma: notes on the management of spoilt identity*. Harmondsworth: Penguin.

Gordon, R. (1988) 'Apartheid's anthropologists: the genealogy of Afrikaner anthropology', *American Ethnologist* 15 (3): 535–53.

Gordon, R. and A. Spiegel (1993) 'Southern Africa revisited', *Annual Review of Anthropology* 22: 83–105.

Government of South Africa (2010) *The National Communications Survey of HIV/AIDS, 2009*. Cape Town: National Government of South Africa. Available at: www.info.gov.za./issues/hiv/survey-

2009.htm#implications (accessed 15 September 2011).

Graham, J., I. Bennett, W. Holmes and R. Gross (2007) 'Medication beliefs as mediators in health literacy: antiretroviral adherence relationship in HIV infected individuals', *AIDS Behaviour* 11: 385–92.

Gussow, Z. and G. Tracy (1977) 'Status, ideology and adaptation to stigmatized illness: a study of leprosy' in D. Landy (ed.), *Culture, Disease and Healing: studies in medical anthropology*. New York NY: Macmillan.

Gutmann, M. (2007) *Fixing Men: sex, birth control and AIDS in Mexico*. Berkeley and Los Angeles CA: University of California Press.

Halperin, D. and R. Bailey (1999) 'Male circumcision and HIV infection: 10 years and counting', *Lancet* 354 (9192): 1813–15.

Hammond-Tooke, W. D. (1981) *Boundaries and Belief: the structure of a Sotho worldview*. Johannesburg: Wits University Press.

— (1989) *Rituals and Medicines: indigenous healing in South Africa*. Johannesburg: A. D. Donker.

Harries, P. (1989) 'Exclusion, classification and internal colonialism: the emergence of ethnicity among Tsonga-speakers of South Africa' in L. Vail (ed.), *The Creation of Tribalism in Southern Africa*. London: James Currey.

Heald, S. (1986) 'The ritual use of violence: circumcision among the Gisu, Uganda' in D. Riches (ed.), *The Anthropology of Violence*. Oxford: Blackwell.

— (1995) 'The power of sex: some reflections on the Caldwells' African sexuality thesis', *Africa* 65 (4): 489–505.

Hecht, T. (1998) *At Home in the Street: street children of northeast Brazil*. Cambridge: Cambridge University Press.

Hellinger, D. (2003) 'Paranoia, conspiracy, and hegemony in

American politics' in H. G. West and T. Sanders (eds), *Transparency and Conspiracy: ethnographies of suspicion in the new world order.* Durham NC and London: Duke University Press.

Helman, C. (1984) 'Disease and pseudo-disease: a case history of pseudo angina' in R. Hahn and S. Gaines (eds), *Physicians of Western Medicine: anthropological perspectives on theory and practice.* Dordrecht: D. Reidel.

— (1994) *Culture, Health and Illness: an introduction for health professionals.* Boston MA: Wright.

— (2006) *Suburban Shaman: tales from medicine's frontline.* London: Hammersmith Press.

— (2014) *An Amazing Murmur of the Heart: feeling the patients' beat.* London: Hammersmith Health Books.

Henderson, P. (2006) 'South African AIDS orphans: examining assumptions around vulnerability from the perspective of rural children and youth', *Childhood* 12 (3): 303–27.

Herring, D. and A. Swelund (2010) *Plagues and Epidemics: infected spaces, past and present.* Oxford: Berg.

Hertz, R. (1960 [1907]) *Death and the Right Hand.* London: Cohen and West.

Hirst, M. (1993) 'The healer's art: Cape Nguni diviners in the townships of Grahamstown, Eastern Cape, South Africa', *Curare* 16 (2): 97–114.

Hlatshwayo, R. (2012) 'Protest over hospital deaths', *The Sowetan,* 17 July. Available at: www. sowetanlive.co.za/news/2012/07/17/ protest-over-hospital-deaths (accessed 20 August 2016).

Hobsbawm, E. and T. Ranger (eds) (1983) *The Invention of Tradition.* Cambridge: Cambridge University Press.

Hollan, D. (2003) 'Self-scape dreams' in J. Mageo (ed.), *Dreaming and the Self: new perspectives on subjectivity, identity and emotion.* New York NY: State University of New York.

Holy, L. (1992) 'Berti dream interpretation' in M. C. Jedrej and R. Shaw (eds), *Dreaming, Religion and Society in Africa.* Leiden: E. J. Brill.

Honwana, A. (2003) 'Undying past: spirit possession and the memory of war in southern Mozambique' in B. Meyer and P. Pels (eds), *Magic and Modernity: interfaces of revelation and concealment.* Stanford CA: Stanford University Press.

Hooper, E. (1999) *The River: a journey to the source of HIV and AIDS.* Boston MA: Little, Brown and Company.

Hull, E. (2017) *Contingent Citizens: professional aspirations in a South African hospital.* London: Bloomsbury.

Hunt, N. (1999) *A Colonial Lexicon of Birth Ritual, Medicalisation and Mobility in the Congo.* Durham NC: Duke University Press.

Hunter, M. (2002) 'The materiality of everyday sex: thinking beyond prostitution', *African Studies* 61 (1): 99–120.

— (2005) 'Cultural politics and masculinities: multiple partners in historical perspective in KwaZulu-Natal' in G. Reid and L. Walker (eds), *Men Behaving Differently: South African men since 1994.* Cape Town: Double Storey.

— (2010) *Love in the Time of AIDS: inequality, gender and rights in South Africa.* Bloomington IN: Indiana University Press.

Hutchinson, S. (1998) 'Death, memory and the politics of legitimation: Nuer experiences of the continuing Sudanese civil war' in R. Werbner (ed.), *Memory and the Postcolony: African anthropology and the critique of power.* London: Zed.

Ibrahim, A. (1994) *Assaulting with Words: popular discourses and the bridle of shar'ia.* Evanston IL: Northwestern University Press.

James, D. (1987) 'Land shortage and inheritance in a Lebowa village', *Social Dynamics* 14 (2): 36–51.

— (1999) *Songs of the Women Migrants: performance and identity in South Africa*. Edinburgh: Edinburgh University Press.

Janzen, J. (1978) *The Quest for Therapy: medical pluralism in Lower Zaire*. Berkeley CA: University of California Press.

Jedrej, M. and R. Shaw (eds) (1992) *Dreaming, Religion and Society in Africa*. Leiden: E. J. Brill.

Jonsson, G. (2004) 'Victim or agent? The construction of young women's sexuality in the South African lowveld'. BA thesis, Department of Anthropology and Archaeology, University of Pretoria.

Kahn, K., M. Garenne, M. Collinson and S. Tollman (2007) 'Mortality rates in the new South Africa: hard to make a fresh start', *Scandinavian Journal of Public Health* 35 (69): 29–34.

Kaler, A. (2001) '"It's some kind of women's empowerment": the ambiguity of the female condom as a marker of female empowerment', *Social Science and Medicine* 52: 783–96.

Kalofonos, I. (2010) '"All I eat is ARVs": the paradox of AIDS treatment interventions in central Mozambique', *Medical Anthropology Quarterly* 24 (3): 363–80.

Kiernan, J. (1994) 'Variations on a Christian theme: the healing synthesis of Zulu Zionism' in R. Shaw and C. Stewart (eds), *Syncretism/Anti-syncretism: the politics of religious synthesis*. London: Routledge.

— (1997) 'Images of rejection in the construction of morality: Satan and the sorcerer as moral signposts in the social landscape of urban Zionists', *Social Anthropology* 5 (2): 243–54.

Killick, E. and A. Desai (2012) 'Introduction: valuing friendship' in A. Desai and E. Killick (eds), *The Ways of Friendship: anthropological perspectives*. New York NY: Berghahn Books.

Klaits, F. (2009) 'Faith and the inter-subjectivity of care in Botswana', *Africa Today* 56 (1): 3–20.

— (2010) *Death in a Church of Life: moral passion during Botswana's time of AIDS*. Berkeley CA: University of California Press.

Kleinman, A. (1978) 'Concepts and a model for comparison of medical systems as cultural systems', *Social Science and Medicine* 12 (1): 85–93.

— (1995) *Writing at the Margin: discourse between anthropology and medicine*. Berkeley CA: University of California Press.

Kluckhohn, C. (1944) *Navaho Witchcraft*. Boston MA: Beacon Press.

Krige, E. J. and J. Krige (1965 [1943]) *The Realm of a Rain Queen*. London: Oxford University Press.

Kroeber, A. (1917) 'The superorganic', *American Anthropologist* 19 (2): 163–213.

Kuper, A. (1982) *Wives for Cattle: bridewealth and marriage in Southern Africa*. London: Routledge.

— (1983) 'The structure of dream sequences', *Culture, Medicine and Psychiatry* 7 (2): 153–75.

— (1994) 'Culture, identity and the project of a cosmopolitan anthropology', *Man* 29 (3): 537–54.

— (2005) *Culture: the anthropologist's account*. Cambridge MA: Harvard University Press.

Lambek, M. (2002) 'Fantasy in practice: projection and introjection, or the witch and the spirit medium' in B. Kapferer (ed.), *Beyond Rationalism: rethinking magic, witchcraft and sorcery*. New York NY: Berghahn Books.

Lane, R. and B. Lane (1959) 'On the development of Dakota-Iroquois and Crow Omaha kinship terminologies', *Southwestern Journal of Anthropology* 15 (3): 254–65.

Langwick, S. (2011) *Bodies, Politics, and African Healing: the matter of maladies in Tanzania*. Bloomington IN: Indiana University Press.

Leclerc-Madlala, S. (1997) '"Infect one, infect all": Zulu responses to the AIDS epidemic in South Africa', *Medical Anthropology* 17 (4): 363–80.

— (2001) 'Virginity testing: managing sexuality in a maturing HIV/AIDS pandemic', *Medical Anthropology Quarterly* 15 (4): 533–52.

— (2002) 'On the virgin cleansing myth: gendered bodies, AIDS and ethnomedicine', *African Journal of AIDS Research* 1 (2): 87–95.

— (2005) 'Popular responses to HIV/AIDS and policy', *Journal of Southern African Studies* 31 (4): 845–56.

— (2006) '"We will eat when I get the grant": negotiating AIDS, poverty and antiretroviral treatment in South Africa', *African Journal of AIDS Research* 5 (3): 249–56.

Lee, R. (2011) 'Death on the move: funerals, entrepreneurship and the rural–urban nexus in South Africa', *Africa* 81 (2): 226–47.

Lee, S. (1958) 'Social influence in Zulu dreaming', *Journal of Social Psychology* 47: 265–83.

Leslie, C. (ed.) (1976) *Asian Medical Systems: a comparative study*. Berkeley CA: University of California Press.

Lévi-Strauss, C. (1963) 'The effectiveness of symbols' in *Structural Anthropology. Volume 1*. New York NY: Basic Books.

Lewis, G. (1987) 'A lesson from Leviticus: leprosy', *Man* 22 (4): 593–612.

LiPuma, E. (1998) 'Modernity and forms of personhood in Melanesia' in M. Lambek and A. Strathern (eds), *Bodies and Persons: comparative perspectives for Africa and Melanesia*. Cambridge: Cambridge University Press.

Livingston, J. (2012) *Improvising Medicine: an African oncology ward in an emerging cancer epidemic*. Durham NC: Duke University Press.

Lubisi, D. (2002) 'South Africa: campaign to deter men from having sex with animals', *African Eye News Service*, 11 April. Available at: http://allafrica. com/stories/200204110545.html (accessed 29 August 2016).

Lupton, D. and A. Petersen (1996) *The New Public Health: health and self in the age of risk*. Thousand Oaks CA: Sage.

MacGregor, H. (2009) 'Mapping the body: tracing the personal and the political dimensions of HIV/AIDS in Khayelitsha, South Africa', *Anthropology and Medicine* 16 (1): 85–95.

MacPherson, P., M. Moshabela, N. Martinson and P. Pronyk (2008) 'Mortality and loss to follow-up among HAART initiators in rural South Africa', *Transactions of the Royal Society for Tropical Medicine and Hygiene* 103 (6): 588–93.

Mageo, J. (2006) 'Figurative dream analysis and US traveling identities', *Ethos* 34 (4): 456–87.

— (2011) *Dreaming Culture: meanings, models and power in US American dreams*. New York NY: St Martins Press.

Mager, A. (2010) *Beer, Sociability and Masculinity in South Africa*. Bloomington IN: Indiana University Press.

Malinowski, B. (1966) *Coral Gardens and their Magic: a study of the methods of tilling the soil and of agricultural rites in the Trobriand islands*. London: Allen and Unwin.

Manona, C. (1980) 'Marriage, family life and migrancy in a Ciskei village' in P. Mayer (ed.), *Black Villagers in an Industrial Society: anthropological perspectives on labour migration in South Africa*. Cape Town: Oxford University Press.

Margaretten, M. (2015) *Street Life under a Roof: youth homelessness in South Africa*. Urbana IL: University of Illinois Press.

Marsland, R. (2012) '(Bio)sociality and HIV in Tanzania: finding a living to support a life', *Medical Anthropology Quarterly* 26 (4): 470–85.

Marsland, R. and R. Prince (2012) 'What is life worth? Exploring biomedical interventions, survival and the politics of life', *Medical Anthropology Quarterly* 26 (4): 453–69.

Martin, E. (1992) *The Woman in the Body: a cultural analysis of reproduction*. Boston MA: Beacon Press.

Mayer, P. and I. Mayer (1970) 'Socialization by peers: the youth organisation of the Red Xhosa' in P. Mayer (ed.), *Socialization: the approach from social anthropology*. London: Routledge.

Mbali, M. (2004) 'AIDS discourses and the South African state: government denialism and post-apartheid policy making', *Transformations* 54: 115–16.

McAllister, P. (1991) 'Using ritual to resist domination in the Transkei', *African Studies* 15 (1): 129–44.

— (2006) *Xhosa Beer Drinking Rituals: power, practice and performance in the South African rural periphery*. Durham NC: Carolina Academic Press.

McNeil, D. (1998) 'Neighbors kill an HIV-positive AIDS activist in South Africa', *New York Times*, 28 December.

McNeill, F. (2009) '"Condoms cause AIDS": poison, prevention and denial in Venda, South Africa', *African Affairs* 108 (432): 353–70.

— (2011) *AIDS, Politics and Music in South Africa*. New York NY: Cambridge University Press.

McNeill, F. and I. Niehaus (2009) *Magic: AIDS review 2009*. Pretoria: Centre for the Study of AIDS, University of Pretoria.

Meinert, L. (2014) 'Regimes of homework in AIDS care: questions of responsibility and the imagination of lives in Uganda' in R. Prince and R. Marsland (eds), *Making and Unmaking Public Health in Africa: ethnographic and historical perspectives*. Athens OH: Ohio University Press.

Meintjes, H. and G. Griese (2006) 'Spinning the epidemic: the making of mythologies of orphanhood in the context of AIDS', *Childhood* 13 (3): 407–30.

Mfecane, S. (2010) 'Exploring masculinities in the context of ARV use: a study of men living with HIV in a South African village'. PhD thesis, WISER, University of the Witwatersrand.

— (2011) 'Negotiating therapeutic citizenship and notions of masculinity in a South African village', *African Journal of AIDS Research* 10 (2): 129–38.

Mitchell, J. (2001) 'Introduction' in P. Clough and J. Mitchell (eds), *Powers of Good and Evil: social transformation and popular belief*. Oxford: Berghahn Books.

Moerman, D. (2002) *Meaning, Medicine and the Placebo Effect*. Cambridge: Cambridge University Press.

Monare, M. (2006) 'Alliance cracks grow as union thrashes call for a woman president', *The Star*, 25 May.

Mönnig, H. O. (1983) *The Pedi*. Pretoria: L. J. Van Schaik.

Murray, C. (1981) *Families Divided: the impact of migrant labour in Lesotho*. Cambridge: Cambridge University Press.

Murray, C. and P. Sanders (2005) *Medicine Murder in Colonial Lesotho: the anatomy of a moral crisis*. Edinburgh: Edinburgh University Press.

Myhre, K. (2009) 'Disease and disruption: Chagga witchcraft and relational fragility' in L. Haram and C. Yamba (eds), *Dealing with Uncertainty in Contemporary African Lives*. Stockholm: Nordiska Afrikainstitutet.

Nachega, J., D. Lehman, D. Hlatshwayo, R. Mothopeng, R. Chaisson and A. Karstaedt (2005) 'HIV/AIDS and antiretroviral treatment knowledge, attitudes, beliefs and practices in HIV-infected adults in Soweto, South Africa', *Journal of Immune Deficiency Syndrome* 38 (2): 196–201.

Natrass, N. (2006) 'South Africa's "rollout" of highly active antiretroviral therapy: a critical assessment', *Journal of Acquired Immune Deficiency Syndromes* 43 (5): 618–23.

— (2007) *Mortal Combat: AIDS denialism and the struggle for antiretrovirals in South Africa.* Pietermaritzburg: University of KwaZulu-Natal Press.

— (2012) *The AIDS Conspiracy: science fights back.* New York NY: Columbia University Press.

Nguyen, V. (2005) 'Antiretroviral globalism: biopolitics, and therapeutic citizenship' in A. Ong and S. Collier (eds), *Global Assemblages: technology, politics, and ethics as anthropological problems.* Oxford: Blackwell.

— (2009) 'Therapeutic evangelism: confessional technologies, antiretrovirals and bio-spiritual transformation in the fight against AIDS in West Africa' in F. Becker and P. W. Geissler (eds), *AIDS and Religious Practice in Africa.* Leiden: Brill.

— (2010) *The Republic of Therapy: triage and sovereignty in West Africa's time of AIDS.* Durham NC: Duke University Press.

Niehaus, I. (1988) 'Domestic dynamics and wage labour: a case study among urban residents in Qwaqwa', *African Studies* 47 (2): 121–43.

— (1993) 'Witch-hunting and political legitimacy: continuity and change in Green Valley, Lebowa, 1930–1991', *Africa* 63 (4): 498–530.

— (1994) 'Disharmonious spouses and harmonious siblings: conceptualizing household formation among urban residents in Qwaqwa', *African Studies* 53 (1): 115–35.

— (1995) 'Witches of the Transvaal lowveld and their familiars: conceptions of duality, power and desire', *Cahiers d'Études Africaines* XXXV-2 (138): 513–40.

— (2000a) 'Towards a dubious liberation: masculinity, sexuality and power in South African lowveld schools, 1953–1999', *Journal of Southern African Studies* 26 (3): 387–407.

— (2000b) 'Coins for blood and blood for coins: from sacrifice to ritual murder in the South African lowveld, 1930–2000', *Etnofoor* 3 (2): 31–54.

— (2002a) 'Ethnicity and the boundaries of belonging: reconfiguring Shangaan identity in the South African lowveld', *African Affairs* 101 (3): 557–83.

— (2002b) 'Bodies, heat and taboos: conceptualising "modern personhood" in the South African lowveld', *Ethnology* 41 (3): 189–207.

— (2002c) 'Perversions of power; witchcraft and the sexuality of evil in the South African lowveld', *Journal of Religion in Africa* 32 (3): 1–31.

— (2005) 'Witches and zombies in the South African lowveld: discourse, accusations and subjective reality', *Journal of the Royal Anthropological Institute* 11 (2): 191–210.

— (2006a) 'Doing politics in Bushbuckridge: work, welfare and the South African elections of 2004', *Africa* 76 (4): 521–48.

— (2006b) 'Biographical lessons: life stories, sex and culture in Bushbuckridge, South Africa', *Cahiers d'Études Africaines* XLVI-1 (181): 51–73.

— (2012a) 'From witch-hunts to thief-hunts: on the temporality of evil in South Africa', *African Historical Review* 44 (1): 29–52.

— (2012b) 'Witchcraft in the South African Bantustans: evidence from Bushbuckridge', *South African Historical Journal* 64 (1): 1–18.

— (2013) *Witchcraft and a Life in the New South Africa*. New York NY: Cambridge University Press.

Niehaus, I. and J. Stadler (2004) '*Muchongolo* dance contests: deep play in the South African lowveld', *Ethnology* 43 (4): 363–80.

Niehaus, I. with E. Mohlala and K. Shokane (2001) *Witchcraft, Power and Politics: exploring the occult in the South African lowveld*. London: Pluto.

Nkuna, W. (1986) 'The contribution and influence of the Holiness Mission churches in the Acornhoek-Bushbuckridge area, 1930–1970'. MA thesis, Department of History, University of South Africa.

Nyamnjoh, F. (2012) 'Blinded by the sight: divining the future of anthropology in Africa', *Africa Spectrum* 47 (2–3): 63–92.

Olsen, W. and C. Sargent (2017) *African Medical Pluralism*. Bloomington IN: Indiana University Press.

Ong, A. and S. Collier (eds) (2005) *Global Assemblages: technology, politics, and ethics as anthropological problems*. Oxford: Blackwell.

Ortner, S. (1984) 'Theory in anthropology since the Sixties', *Comparative Studies in Society and History* 26 (1): 126–66.

Oxlund, B. (2009) *Love in Limpopo: becoming a man in a South African university campus*. PhD series no. 54. Copenhagen: Department of Anthropology, University of Copenhagen.

Parker, R. and P. Aggleton (2003) 'HIV and AIDS-related stigma and discrimination: a conceptual framework and implications for action', *Social Science and Medicine* 57 (1): 13–24.

Pawninski, R. and U. Lalloo (2001) 'Community attitudes to HIV/AIDS', *South African Medical Journal* 91: 448–53.

Peek, P. (1991) 'African divination systems: non-normal modes of cognition' in P. M. Peek (ed.), *African Divination Systems: ways of knowing*. Bloomington IN: Indiana University Press.

Peterson, K. (2014) *Speculative Markets: drug companies and derivative life in Nigeria*. Durham NC: Duke University Press.

Petryna, A. (2002) *Life Exposed: biological citizens after Chernobyl*. Princeton NJ: Princeton University Press.

— (2004) 'Biological citizenship: the science and politics of Chernobyl-exposed populations', *Osiris* 19: 250–65.

— (2009) *When Experiments Travel: clinical trials and the global search for human subject*. Princeton NJ: Princeton University Press.

Petryna, A., A. Lakoff and A. Kleinman (eds) (2006) *global pharmaceuticals: ethics, markets, practices*. Raleigh NC: Duke University Press.

Peyper, L. (2017) 'Unemployment at record high for third quarter in a row', *News24*, 31 October. Available at: www.fin24.com/Economy/unemployment-at-record-high-for-third-quarter-in-a-row-20171031 (accessed 6 November 2017).

Pigg, S. (2001) 'Languages of sex and AIDS in Nepal: notes on the social production of commensurability', *Cultural Anthropology* 16 (4): 481–541.

Posel, D. (2005) 'Sex, death and the fate of the nation: reflections on the politicization of sexuality in post-apartheid South Africa', *Africa* 75 (2): 125–53.

Prince, R. (2013) 'Introduction: situating health and the public in Africa' in R. Prince and R. Marsland (eds), *Making and Unmaking Public Health in Africa: ethnographic and historical perspectives*. Athens OH: Ohio University Press.

Probst, P. (1999) 'Mchape '95, or, the sudden fame of Billy Goodson Chisupe: healing, social memory and the enigma of the public sphere in post-Banda Malawi', *Africa* 69 (1): 108–38.

Pronyk, P. (2001) 'Assessing health-seeking behaviour among tuberculosis patients in rural South Africa', *International Journal of Tuberculosis and Lung Disease* 5 (7): 619–27.

Rabinow, P. and N. Rose (2006) 'Biopower today', *BioSocieties* 1: 195–217.

Radcliffe-Brown, A. R. (1950) 'Introduction' in A. R. Radcliffe-Brown and C. D. Forde (eds), *African Systems of Kinship and Marriage*. London: Oxford University Press.

— (1952a) 'The mother's brother in South Africa' in *Structure and Function in Primitive Society*. London: Cohen and West.

— (1952b) 'On joking relationships' in *Structure and Function in Primitive Society*. London: Cohen and West.

Reynolds Whyte, S. (ed.) (2014) *Second Chances: surviving AIDS in Uganda*. Durham NC: Duke University Press.

Robins, S. (2004) '"Long live Zackie, long live": AIDS activism, science and citizenship after apartheid', *Journal of Southern African Studies* 30 (3): 651–72.

— (2006) 'From "rights" to "ritual": AIDS activism in South Africa', *American Anthropologist* 108 (2): 312–23.

Rose, N. (2001) 'The politics of life itself', *Theory, Culture and Society* 18 (1): 1–30.

— (2006) *The Politics of Life Itself: biomedicine, power, and subjectivity in the twenty-first century*. Princeton NJ: Princeton University Press.

Rose, N. and C. Novas (2005) 'Biological citizenship' in A. Ong and S. Collier (eds), *Global Assemblages: technology, politics and*

ethics as anthropological problems. Oxford: Blackwell.

Rosenberg, C. (1992) *Explaining Epidemics and Other Studies in the History of Medicine*. Cambridge: Cambridge University Press.

Sahlins, M. (1985) *Islands of History*. Chicago IL and London: University of Chicago Press.

— (1993) 'Goodbye to *tristes tropes*: ethnography in the context of modern world history', *Journal of Modern History* 65 (1): 1–25.

— (1999) 'Two or three things that I know about culture', *Journal of the Royal Anthropological Institute* 5 (3): 399–421.

— (2004) *Apologies to Thucydides: understanding history as culture and vice versa*. Chicago IL: University of Chicago Press.

SAIRR (1988). *South African Survey 1987/1988*. Johannesburg: South African Institute of Race Relations (SAIRR).

— (2001) *South African Survey 2000/2001*. Johannesburg: South African Institute of Race Relations (SAIRR).

Sanders, T. and H. West (2003) 'Power revealed and concealed in the new world order' in H. G. West and T. Sanders (eds), *Transparency and Conspiracy: ethnographies of suspicion in the new world order*. Durham NC and London: Duke University Press.

Sartre, J.-P. (1960) *Critique de la raison dialectique précédé de Questions de méthode*. Paris: Gallimard.

Schatz, E. and C. Ogunmefun (2007) 'Caring and contributing: the role of older women in rural South African multi-generational households with AIDS', *World Development* 35 (8): 1390–403.

Scheffler, H. (2001) 'Remuddling kinship: the state of the art', *Zeitschrift für Ethnologie* 126 (2): 161–74

Schenker, I. (2006) *HIV/AIDS Literacy: an essential component in Education for All*. EFA Global

Monitoring Report. Paris: UNESCO.

Schneider, D. (1968) *American Kinship: a cultural account*. Chicago IL: University of Chicago Press.

Schneider, H. and D. Fassin (2002) 'Denial and defiance: a socio-political analysis of AIDS in South Africa', *AIDS* 16 (2): 1–7.

Schoepf, B. (1988) 'Women, AIDS and economic crisis in Central Africa', *Canadian Journal of African Studies* 22 (3): 625–44.

— (2001) 'International AIDS research in anthropology: taking a critical perspective on the crisis', *Annual Review of Anthropology* 61: 335–61.

Schumaker, L. (2001) *Africanizing Anthropology: fieldwork, networks and the making of cultural knowledge in Central Africa*. Durham NC: Duke University Press.

Scorgie, F. (2002) 'Virginity testing and the politics of sexual responsibility: implications for AIDS intervention', *African Studies* 61 (1): 55–75.

Scott, J. (1990) *Domination and the Arts of Resistance: hidden transcripts*. New Haven CT: Yale University Press.

Scott, M. (2007) *The Severed Snake: matri-lineages, making place, and a Melanesian Christianity in Southeast Solomon Islands*. Durham NC: Carolina Academic Press.

Segalen, M. (1984) 'Nuclear is not independent: organization of the household in Pays Bigouden Sud in the nineteenth and twentieth centuries' in R. McC. Netting, R. Wilk and E. Arnould (eds), *Households: comparative and historical studies of the domestic group*. Berkeley CA: University of California Press.

Senah, K. (1994) '*Blofo Tshofa*: local perceptions of medicines in a Ghanaian coastal community' in N. Etkin and M. Tan (eds), *Medicines: meanings and contexts*. Quezon City PA: Health Action Information Network.

Setel, P. (1999) *A Plague of Paradoxes: AIDS, culture and demography in northern Tanzania*. Chicago IL and London: University of Chicago Press.

Sharp, J. and A. Spiegel (1985) 'Vulnerability to impoverishment in South African rural areas: the erosion of kinship and neighbourhood as social resources', *Africa* 55 (2): 133–52.

Shaw, R. and C. Stewart (1994) 'Introduction: problematizing syncretism' in R. Shaw and C. Stewart (eds), *Syncretism/Anti-syncretism: the politics of religious synthesis*. London: Routledge.

Shell, R. (2001) 'Trojan horses: HIV/AIDS and military bases in Southern Africa'. Paper presented to the AIDS in Context conference, University of the Witwatersrand, Johannesburg, 4–7 April.

Shisana, O. et al. (2002) *Nelson Mandela/HSRC Study of HIV/AIDS*. Cape Town: Human Sciences Research Council Press.

Silla, E. (1998) *People are Not the Same: leprosy and insanity in twentieth-century Mali*. Portsmouth NH: Heinemann.

Singer, M. (1989) 'The coming age of critical medical anthropology', *Social Science and Medicine* 28 (11): 1193–203.

Skhosana, N. (2001) 'Women, HIV/AIDS and stigma: an anthropological study of life in a hospice'. MA thesis, University of the Witwatersrand.

Skhosana, N., H. Struthers. G. Gray and J. McIntyre (2006) 'HIV disclosure and other factors that impact adherence to antiretroviral therapy: the case of Soweto, South Africa', *African Journal of AIDS Research* 5 (1): 17–26.

Sobo, E. J. (1993) 'Inner-city women and AIDS: the psycho-social benefits of unsafe sex', *Culture, Medicine and Psychiatry* 17 (4): 455–85.

South African Medical Research Council (2015) *Rapid Mortality*

Surveillance Report 2013. Pretoria: Government Printers.

Spiegel, A. (1986) 'Dispersing dependants: a response to the exigencies of migrant labour in rural Transkei' in J. Eades (ed.), *Migrants, Workers and the Social Order*. London: Tavistock.

— (1989) 'Polygyny as myth: towards understanding extramarital relations in Lesotho' in A. Spiegel and P. McAllister (eds), *Tradition and Transition in Southern Africa*. Johannesburg: Witwatersrand University Press.

Stadler, J. (1994) 'Generational relationships in a lowveld village: questions of age, household, and tradition'. MA thesis, Department of Social Anthropology, University of the Witwatersrand.

— (2003a) 'The young, the rich and the beautiful: secrecy, suspicion and discourses of AIDS in the South African lowveld', *African Journal of AIDS Research* 2 (2): 127–39.

— (2003b) 'Rumour, gossip and blame: implications of HIV/AIDS prevention in the South African lowveld', *AIDS Education and Prevention* 15 (4): 357–69.

— (2011) 'Shared secrets – concealed sufferings: social responses to the AIDS epidemic in Bushbuckridge, South Africa'. PhD thesis, University of Pretoria.

Stadler, J. and L. Hlongwa (2002) 'Monitoring and evaluation of LoveLife's AIDS prevention and advocacy activities in South Africa, 1999–2001', *Evaluation and Program Planning* 25 (2): 365–76.

Staff Reporter (2003) 'Dog rape: strict bail conditions', *News24 Archives*, 4 October. Available at: www.news24.com/SouthAfrica/News/Dog-rape-Strict-bail-conditions-20030410 (accessed 29 August 2016).

Stein, J. (2003) 'HIV/AIDS stigma: the latest dirty secret', *African Journal of AIDS Research* 2 (2): 95–101.

Steinberg, J. (2008) *Three Letter Plague: a young man's journey through a great epidemic*. Johannesburg and Cape Town: Jonathan Ball.

Steven, M., A. Cockroft, G. Lamothe and N. Andersson (2010) 'Equity in HIV testing: evidence from a cross-sectional study in ten South African countries', *International Health and Human Rights* 10 (23): 67–89.

Stoler, A. (1995) *Race and the Education of Desire: Foucault's History of Sexuality and the Colonial Order of Things*. Durham NC: Duke University Press.

Strathern, M. (1996) 'Cutting the network', *Journal of the Royal Anthropological Institute* 2 (3): 517–35.

Street, A. (2014) *Biomedicine in an Unstable Place: infrastructure and personhood in a Papua New Guinea hospital*. Durham NC: Duke University Press.

Sundkler, B. (1961) *Bantu Prophets in South Africa*. London: Oxford University Press.

Tambiah, S. (1968) 'The magical power of words', *Man* 3 (2): 175–208.

Taussig, M. (1980) 'Reification and consciousness of the patient', *Social Science and Medicine* 14 (1): 3–13.

Taylor, C. (1992) *Milk, Honey and Money: changing concepts in Rwandan healing*. Washington DC: Smithsonian Institution Press.

Thomas, L. (2009) 'Love, sex, and the modern girl in 1930s Southern Africa' in J. Cole and L. M. Thomas (eds), *Love in Africa*. Chicago IL: University of Chicago Press.

Thomas, N. (1992) 'The inversion of tradition', *American Ethnologist* 19 (1): 213–32.

Thornton, R. (2008) *Unimagined Community: sex, networks and AIDS in Uganda and in South Africa*. Berkeley CA: University of California Press.

— (2017) *Healing the Exposed Being: the Ngoma healing tradition in South Africa.* Johannesburg: Wits University Press.

Tollman, S., K. Kahn, K. Herbst, M. Garenne and J. Gear (1999) 'Reversal in mortality trends: evidence from the Agincourt field site, South Africa, 1992 to 1999', *AIDS* 13: 1091–7.

Townsend, N. (1997) 'Men, migration and households in Botswana: an exploration of connections over time and space', *Journal of Southern African Studies* 23 (3): 405–20.

Treichler, P. (1999) *How to Have Theory in an Epidemic: cultural chronicles of AIDS.* Durham NC: Duke University Press.

Tsing, A. (2004) *Friction: an ethnography of global connection.* Princeton NJ: Princeton University Press.

Turner, V. (1967) *The Forest of Symbols.* Ithaca NY: Cornell University Press.

Twine, R., M. A. Collinson, T. J. Polzer and K. Kahn (2007) 'Evaluating access to a child-oriented poverty alleviation intervention in rural South Africa', *Scandinavian Journal of Public Health* 35 (69): 118–27.

Tylor, E. (1958 [1871]) *Primitive Culture. Volume 2: The origin of religion.* New York NY: Harper Torchbooks.

Van der Geest, S. (2006) 'Between death and funeral: mortuaries and the exploitation of liminality in Kwahu, Ghana', *Africa* 76 (4): 485–501.

Van der Geest, S. and A. Hardon (2003) *Social Lives of Medicines.* Cambridge: Cambridge University Press.

Van der Geest, S., S. Reynolds Whyte and A. Hardon (1996) 'The anthropology of pharmaceuticals: a biographical approach', *Annual Review of Anthropology* 25: 153–78.

Van der Vliet, V. (1991) 'Traditional husbands, modern wives: constructing marriage in an African township' in A. Spiegel and P. McAllister (eds), *Tradition and Transition in Southern Africa.* Johannesburg: Witwatersrand University Press.

Van Wyk, I. (2012) 'A response', *Anthropology Southern Africa* 35 (3–4): 119–21.

Vaughan, M. (1991) *Curing their Ills: colonial power and African illness.* Cambridge: Polity Press.

Versteeg, M., M. Heywood, T. Maseko and D. Kegakilwe (2013) 'No improvement in Tintswalo hospital prompts open letter to Mpumalanga Department of Health', SANGONet, 29 August. Available at: www.ngopulse.org/press-release/no-improvement-tintswalo-hospital-prompts-open-letter-mpumalanga-department-health (accessed 27 August 2016).

Viljoen, F. (2005) 'Disclosing in the age of AIDS: confidentiality and community in conflict' in F. Viljoen (ed.), *Righting Stigma: exploring a rights-based approach to addressing stigma.* Pretoria: Human Rights Research Unit, University of Pretoria.

Wahlstrom, Å. (2002) 'The old digging graves for the young: the cultural construction of AIDS among youth in the South African lowveld'. BSc thesis, Brunel University, London.

Ware, N., J. Idoko, S. Kaaya, I. Biraro, M. Wyatt, O. Agbaji, G. Chalamilla and D. Bangsberg (2009) 'Explaining adherence success in sub-Saharan Africa: an ethnographic study', *Plos Medicine* 6 (1): 39–47.

Webster, D. (1977) 'Spreading the risk: the principle of laterality among the Chopi', *Africa* 47 (2): 192–207.

Weckesser, A. (2011) 'Girls, gifts and gender: an ethnography of maternal care in rural Mpumalanga, South Africa'. PhD thesis, School of Health and Social

Studies, University of Warwick.

Weiss, B. (1993) 'Buying her grave: money, movement and AIDS in northwest Tanzania', *Africa* 63 (1): 19–35.

West, H. (2007) *Ethnographic Sorcery*. Chicago IL: University of Chicago Press.

Weston, K. (1997) *Families We Choose: lesbians, gays, kinship*. New York NY: Columbia University Press.

White, L. (2000) *Speaking with Vampires: rumour and history in colonial Africa*. Berkeley CA: University of California Press.

Whyte, M. (2013) 'Episodic fieldwork, updating and sociability', *Social Analysis* 57 (1): 110–21.

Wilson, M. (1951) 'Witch beliefs and social structure', *American Journal of Sociology* 56 (4): 307–13.

Wojcicki, J. (2002) '"She drank his money": survival sex and the problem of violence in taverns in Gauteng Province, South Africa', *Medical Anthropology Quarterly* 16 (3): 267–93.

Wolf, E. (1982) *Europe and the People without History*. Berkeley and Los Angeles CA: University of California Press.

Wood, K. and H. Lambert (2008) 'Coded talk, scripted omissions: the micro-politics of AIDS talk in an affected community in South Africa', *Medical Anthropology Quarterly* 22 (3): 213–33.

Yamba, B. (1997) 'Cosmologies in turmoil: witch-finding and AIDS in Chiawa, Zambia', *Africa* 67 (2): 200–23.

Zhang, E. (2007) 'Switching between traditional Chinese medicine and Viagra: cosmopolitanism and medical pluralism today', *Medical Anthropology* 26 (1): 53–96.

Zwang, J., M. Garenne, K. Kahn, M. Collinson and S. Tollman (2007) 'Trends in mortality from pulmonary tuberculosis and HIV/AIDS co-infection in rural South Africa (Agincourt)', *Transactions of the Royal Society of Tropical Medicine and Hygiene* 101 (9): 893–98.

Index

Note: Page numbers followed by n indicate a footnote with relevant number.

Mobility between Africa, Asia and Latin America: Economic Networks and Cultural Interactions
EDITED BY UTE RÖSCHENTHALER AND ALESSANDRO JEDLOWSKI

'Empirically rich and conceptually astute, this volume gives the reader unparalleled insight into the lives of mobile traders crisscrossing the Global South. Essential reading for anyone interested in contemporary globalization and its historical roots.'

Neil Carrier, University of Oxford

'This important collection offers compelling accounts of geopolitical histories, personal trajectories, and unexpected cultural outcomes. The volume is recommended to anyone interested in Africa's diverse transnational connections.'

Heidi Østbø Haugen, University of Oslo

Agricultural Reform in Rwanda: Authoritarianism, Markets and Zones of Governance
BY CHRIS HUGGINS

'A very informed, nuanced analysis of agriculture in Rwanda, spanning zones of governance, compliance and resistance in a "developmental" state. As always, only some citizens and communities benefit. This book shows us why.'

Timothy M. Shaw, University of Massachusetts Boston

'An extraordinary study of the state-directed commercialization of Rwandan agriculture. In this nuanced account, Huggins reworks the contemporary agrarian question.'

Philip McMichael, Cornell University